Myocardial
Laser
Revascularization

I would like to thank Libby Deluca, my erstwhile secretary, who moved on to greener pastures and greater responsibility in her career. Yet she remained committed to this project to its completion, offering graciously to continue to volunteer her continuing efforts on our behalf. Without her hard work this would not have been possible.
CB

All of us want to thank our families, Renee, Hillary, Amanda, and Lauren (CB); Hallie, Hanna, Hazel, and Cathy (KH); and Jane Mong-Hua (RC), for their tolerance of our sometimes overbearing work ethic and to let each of you know that without your love and support we could never have been successful in this project.
CB, KH, RC

Myocardial Laser Revascularization

Edited by

Charles R. Bridges, MD ScD

Chief of Cardiothoracic Surgery
Pennsylvania Hospital
Associate Professor of Surgery
University of Pennsylvania Medical Center
Philadelphia, PA
USA

Keith A. Horvath, MD

Chief, Cardiothoracic Surgery Branch
National Heart, Lung and Blood Institute, NIH
Bethesda, MD
USA

Ray Chu-Jeng Chiu, MD PhD FRCSC

Professor of Surgery and Chair Emeritus
McGill University
Montreal General Hospital
Montreal, Quebec
Canada

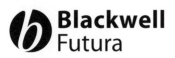

Blackwell
Futura

© 2006 by Blackwell Publishing
Blackwell Futura is an imprint of Blackwell Publishing

Blackwell Publishing, Inc., 350 Main Street, Malden, Massachusetts 02148-5020, USA
Blackwell Publishing Ltd, 9600 Garsington Road, Oxford OX4 2DQ, UK
Blackwell Science Asia Pty Ltd, 550 Swanston Street, Carlton, Victoria 3053, Australia

First published 2006

1   2006

ISBN-13: 978-1-4051-2210-8
ISBN-10: 1-4051-2210-2

Library of Congress Cataloging-in-Publication Data

Myocardial laser revascularization / edited by Charles Bridges, Keith A. Horvath, Ray Chu-Jeng Chiu.
    p. ; cm.
    Includes bibliographical references and index.
    ISBN-13: 978-1-4051-2210-8 (alk. paper)
    ISBN-10: 1-4051-2210-2 (alk. paper)
    1. Myocardial revascularization.   2. Lasers in surgery.
    [DNLM: 1. Myocardial Revascularization.   2. Laser Surgery. WG 169 M9966 2006]
I. Bridges, Charles, 1956–   II. Horvath, Keith A.   III. Chiu, Ray Chu-Jeng.

    RD598.35.M95M96   2006
    617.4'120598 — dc22

                                                                      2006004376

A catalogue record for this title is available from the British Library

Set in 9.5/12pt Palatino by SNP Best-set Typesetter Ltd., Hong Kong
Printed and bound in India by Replika Press Pvt., Ltd

Acquisitions: Steve Korn
Development Editor: Simone Dudziak
Production Controller: Kate Charman

For further information on Blackwell Publishing, visit our website:
www.blackwellcardiology.com

Notice: The indications and dosages of all drugs in this book have been recommended in the medical literature and conform to the practices of the general community. The medications described do not necessarily have specific approval by the Food and Drug Administration for use in the diseases and dosages for which they are recommended. The package insert for each drug should be consulted for use and dosage as approved by the FDA. Because standards for usage change, it is advisable to keep abreast of revised recommendations, particularly those concerning new drugs.

Contents

List of Contributors

Keith B. Allen, MD
Cardiac Surgeon
Department of Cardiothoracic Surgery
CORVASC, MDs
Indianapolis, IN
USA

John Andrew Armour, MD PhD
Associate Professor
Department of Pharmacology
University of Montreal
Montreal, Quebec
Canada

Marianne Bergheim, BA
Research Assistant
The University of Texas
Health Science Center
Houston, TX
USA

Charles R. Bridges, MD ScD
Chief of Cardiothoracic Surgery
Pennsylvania Hospital
Associate Professor of Surgery
University of Pennsylvania Medical Center
Philadephia, PA
USA

Ray Chu-Jeng Chiu, MD PhD FRCSC
Professor of Surgery and Chair Emeritus
McGill University
Montreal General Hospital
Montreal, Quebec
Canada

Chad E. Darling, MD
Assistant Professor of Emergency Medicine
University of Massachusetts Medical School
Worcester, MA
USA

O.H. Frazier, MD
Chief, Cardiopulmonary Transplantation
Director, Cardiovascular Surgery Research
Texas Heart Institute
Houston, TX
USA

Kapil Gopal, MD
Department of Surgery
Lennox Hill Hospital
New York, NY
USA

Keith A. Horvath, MD
Chief, Cardiothoracic Surgery Branch
National Heart, Lung and Blood Institute, NIH
Bethesda, MD
USA

G. Chad Hughes, MD
Assistant Professor
Division of Thoracic and Cardiovascular Surgery
Duke University Medical Center
Durham, NC
USA

E. Duco Jansen, PhD
Associate Professor of Biomedical Engineering
Associate Professor of Neurosurgery
Department of Biomedical Engineering
Vanderbilt University
Nashville, TN
USA

Kamuran A. Kadipasaoglu, PhD
Assistant Director
Cardiovascular Surgical Research Laboratories
Texas Heart Institute
Houston, TX
USA

Varun Kapila, PhD
University of Ottawa
Faculty of Medicine
Ottawa, Ontario
Canada

Stephen J. Korkola, MD, FRCSC
Cardiac Surgeon
Regina General Hospital
Regina, Saskatchewan
Canada

Kevin Lachapelle, MD, FRCSC
Associate Professor of Surgery
Division of Cardiac Surgery
McGill University Health Centre
Montreal, Quebec
Canada

James E. Lowe, MD
Professor of Surgery
Duke University Medical Center
Durham, NC
USA

Marc P. Pelletier, MD, MSc, FRCSC
Assistant Professor
Department of Thoracic Surgery
Stanford University
Mountain View, CA
USA

Egemen Tuzun, MD
Research Scientist
Cardiovascular Surgical Research Laboratories
Texas Heart Institute
Houston, TX
USA

Peter Whittaker, PhD
Associate Professor of Emergency Medicine &
    Anesthesiology
Department of Emergency Medicine
University of Massachusetts Medical School
Worcester, MA
USA

Preface

Completeness of revascularization has long been a mainstay of the surgical treatment of coronary artery disease. This goal has become increasingly difficult with a marked rise in the number of patients that have severe diffuse coronary artery disease. While percutaneous interventions have certainly been successful in treating coronary lesions their impact has been to further skew the population of patients that are referred for surgery and stenting is also limited by diffuse coronary disease.

With these limitations of conventional revascularization, novel methods to improve myocardial blood flow and perfusion have been investigated. One of these methods that has demonstrated clinical success is transmyocardial laser revascularization (TMR). Initially based teleologically on the idea of the reptilian heart in which blood flows directly from the left ventricle into the myocardium, laser channels were created to mimic similar direct pathways. Experimental work has indicated that the principal mechanism for TMR may be the stimulation of new blood vessels rather than the creation of transmural channels. TMR has been demonstrated in multiple randomized controlled trials to provide symptom relief for patients with severe angina. Based on these findings with sole therapy TMR, combination use with coronary artery bypass grafting has also been performed.

The intent of this book is to provide the reader with a complete understanding of the indications, results, mechanisms, and limitations of transmyocardial laser revascularization. While our understanding and treatment of the macrocirculation of the heart is reasonably well understood, our grasp of the micro-circulation as evidenced by the clinical success of TMR is less axiomatic.

Charles Bridges
Keith Horvath
Ray Chiu
2006

CHAPTER 1

Scientific and historic precedents

OH Frazier, Marianne Bergheim, and Kamuran A Kadipasaoglu

Introduction

Transmyocardial laser revascularization (TMR) is based on anatomic and physiologic principles long known and accepted in the history of medicine. The coronary anatomy was first described accurately by Vesalius in his landmark
16th-century text, *De humani corporis fabrica* [1]. The anatomic pathway of the
coronary circulation was further elucidated by Vieussens [2], the royal physician to Louis XIV [3]. Vieussens documented the presence of direct vascular
communication between coronary arteries and the chambers of the heart [4]. In
1706, he published *Nouvelles découvertes sur le coeur*, which was recognized at the
time as the most accurate and detailed account of the structure and function of
the heart [5]. This work described the circulation of the heart as inferred from
postmortem experiments on the hearts of humans, calves, and sheep [2,3].
In these studies, Vieussens ligated the vena cava and pulmonary veins and injected saffron dye dissolved in alcohol into the coronary arteries. Once injected,
the dye solution not only followed the accepted anatomic conduit through the
coronary sinus and into the right atrium, but also flowed directly into the right
and left ventricular chambers through small channels in the walls of the atria
and ventricles [6]. Vieussens labeled these ducts joining the ventricular cavities
to the coronary arteries "ducti carnosi" [2,4].

Two years later in Leiden, Holland, Thebesius [7] published *De circulo sanguinis in corde*, also relating to the microanatomy of the myocardium. Thebesius discovered openings in the endocardium by injecting water into the coronary sinus
and observing the subsequent arrival of effluent in the atria and ventricles. Further experiments in which air, colored liquids mixed with wax, and glue were
injected into the coronary veins provided the same results, confirming the
presence of the ducts in the cardiac chambers [4,6]. Thebesius and Vieussens described the same channels, Thebesius by injecting the veins and Vieussens by injecting the arteries. Although Vieussens first reported the existence of these
openings, all myocardial vessels that connect to cardiac chambers are now
called thebesian vessels. In any case, by the early 18th century, the unique character of the coronary circulation was well established.

The study of comparative anatomy was popularized by the French anatomist
Cuvier [8] in the late 18th and early 19th centuries. Cuvier described various
ways that nature dealt with the problem of vascularizing the organ responsible

for supplying blood to the rest of the body. As one moves up the evolutionary ladder, the circulation moves from one of direct perfusion from the ventricular cavity through the spongy, non-compacted myocardium as seen in fish and reptiles to one of direct coronary blood flow as seen in mammals. Interestingly, the various steps in this phylogenetic evolution of the coronary circulation are closely recapitulated in the development of the human embryo. Historically, the presence of this retained non-compacted myocardium contributing to a pathologic condition was first noted by Grant [9] in the 1920s. This abnormality, which may be seen in both symptomatic and asymptomatic patients [10,11], is appreciated more today because of the precise diagnostic capabilities of cardiac magnetic resonance imaging (MRI) and echocardiography.

The physiologic potential and possible functional importance of this direct ventriculomyocardial communication was demonstrated by a simple, yet ingenious, experiment by Pratt [12] in 1898. Pratt demonstrated that, by delivering defibrinated blood directly into the ventricular cavity and totally excluding the coronary circulation, it was still possible to maintain cardiac contractility and function, with the only source of oxygenated blood being directly through the ventricular myocardium. In this way, contractility was maintained in a mammalian model for several hours (Figure 1.1).

In 1928, while working in Boston's city morgue, Leary and Wearn [13] detailed the postmortem coronary circulation in two patients who had chronic syphilitic aortitis. Syphilitic aortitis had long been known to selectively invade the ascending aorta. In these two patients, the aortic origin of both coronary arteries had been chronically occluded by this disease. In spite of this, both patients were known to have maintained active lifestyles and gainful employment for a number of years before they died. This finding particularly intrigued Wearn and moved him to question how blood was able to reach the heart despite the obliteration of the coronary access.

After relocating to Western Reserve University in Cleveland, Wearn [6] embarked on a study to further elucidate this question. He studied human hearts by perfusing the coronary arteries with a celloidin mass too thick to enter the capillaries and subsequently observed celloidin plugs in the walls of the heart chambers, indicating that the celloidin had bypassed the capillaries. He detailed his findings in a paper published in 1933 [6]. Dissection and negative casting revealed direct vascular communication between the coronary arteries and the ventricular cavities via two types of vessels, identified as the arterioluminal and arteriosinusoidal vessels. Located near the endocardium, the arterioluminal vessels run directly from the coronary arteries into the lumen of the heart. The arteriosinusoidal vessels are small branches of coronary arteries that eventually lose their arterial character and divide into channels called myocardial sinusoids (Figure 1.2). Myocardial sinusoids vary in diameter from 50 to 250 µm and have thin walls consisting of endothelial tissue.

The study of myocardial circulation became much more pertinent throughout the 1920s and into the 1930s, as angina and coronary artery disease in general became increasingly observed clinically. Nevertheless, the treatment

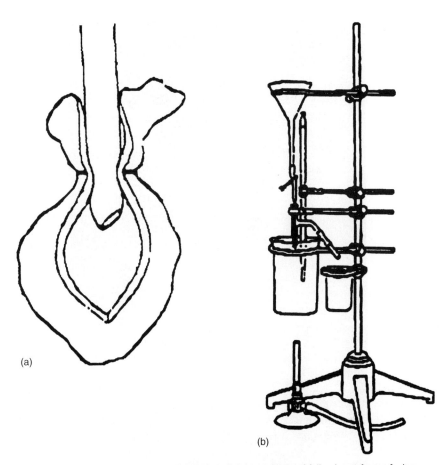

Figure 1.1 (a) Diagram illustrating cannulation of right ventricle of feline heart for perfusion through thebesian veins. (b) This apparatus perfused the feline heart with defibrinated blood through the ventricles and maintained myocardial contractility for several hours. From Pratt [12] with permission.

options for coronary artery disease in this era were limited to symptomatic therapies such as nitroglycerin, which reduced or palliated anginal symptoms.

Claude Beck [14–20], who had been a surgeon in Boston and had also moved to Western Reserve University School of Medicine in Cleveland, was aware of the work of Wearn and was intrigued by his observations regarding the microcirculation of the heart. Beck had also observed extensive collateral blood supply accompanying the restrictive pericarditis frequently associated with tuberculosis. To Beck this seemed to imply that augmentation of blood supply was being induced by an inflammatory response to this infectious process. The possibility implied by Wearn's work was that this augmented blood supply might reach the myocardium directly, thereby bypassing the occluded coronary arteries. Beck attempted to produce this response by irritating the myocardium through abrasion and introduction of foreign bodies (talc) [14,15].

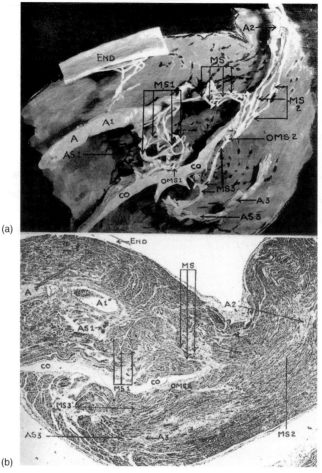

(a)

(b)

Figure 1.2 (a) Wax reconstruction revealing direct communication between coronary arteries and left ventricle via arterioluminal and arteriosinusoidal vessels. (b) Serial section from block of myocardium used to create the wax reconstruction shown in top panel (magnification ×41). A, artery; AS, arteriosinusoidal vessel; CO, common opening; END, endocardium; MS, myocardial sinusoid; OMS, opening of a myocardial sinusoid into ventricular lumen. From Wearn et al. [6] with permission.

The historic demonstrations of Vieussens and Thebesius implied that direct arterial blood could be brought to the ischemic myocardium by utilizing the venous system. Beck decided to bring arterial blood to the ischemic myocardium in the same way. This approach was once again based on the extensive interconnecting microcirculatory network that proliferated in response to myocardial ischemia. Beck utilized the brachial artery as a graft and the coronary sinus as a conduit from the descending aorta. This operation was researched extensively in the experimental animal and first applied to patients in 1948 [17]. The intrepid Beck performed this milestone operation without benefit of today's modern vascular instruments or suture materials and, more important-ly, without access to cardiopulmonary bypass. This retrograde bypass was per-formed 20 years before the introduction of antegrade coronary artery bypass procedures. Beck combined various approaches to this indirect revasculariza-tion, utilizing chemical and mechanical means to enhance anastomotic channels through adhesions combined, in some cases, with arterialization of the coronary sinus [14–20]. Despite a high mortality rate for these procedures, Beck reported relief of anginal symptoms in the majority of patients [17–20].

Taking an even more direct approach to myocardial revascularization, the Canadian surgeon Vineberg [21,22] began implanting the internal mammary artery (IMA) into the left ventricular wall of canine hearts in 1945. This direct myocardial revascularization technique took advantage of the sponge-like character of the myocardial sinusoids, thus allowing direct communication between the IMA implant and myocardial cells. Postoperative studies con-firmed microscopic anastomosis between the open IMA graft and the arteriolar branches of the poorly functioning canine coronary artery. Vineberg performed this procedure for the first time on a patient with coronary insufficiency in 1950 [22]. The majority of patients reported improvement in anginal symptoms as well as increased duration of physical activity. Vineberg's angiographic demon-stration of the patency of the open IMA graft, as well as extensive communica-tion to the microcirculation of the heart, enhanced the credibility of these anecdotal reports. The introduction of cardiopulmonary bypass, as well as im-provements in vascular instruments and suture materials, allowed coronary artery bypass grafting (CABG) to supplant the Vineberg procedure by the late 1960s. Nevertheless, in 1975, Vineberg [23] demonstrated the long-term effec-tiveness of the IMA graft procedure when he reported the continued patency of the arteriomyocardial connections and the important symptomatic relief afforded by the procedure after 24 years of follow-up (Figure 1.3). The report included 94 patients, with 84% showing graft patency.

Following Goldman *et al.*'s proposal [24] in 1957 to create a direct communi-cation between the ventricular cavity and coronary circulation using straight and U-shaped arterial grafts, Massimo and Boffi [25] initiated the use of T-shaped polyethylene tubes to offer more protection against obstruction caused by compression during myocardial contractions. That same year, Massimo and Boffi reported that the T-shaped tubes successfully delivered oxygenated blood from the left ventricle directly into the ischemic myocardium of dogs.

In 1964, before CABG had become generally accepted, Sen *et al.* [26–28] re-ported the use of a unique method of direct revascularization. They based their approach on the accepted corollary, established by Wearn, Pratt, Vineberg, and others, that myocardial viability is preserved by the proliferation of the micro-circulation. The aim was to enhance blood flow to the ischemic myocardium by creating small channels with a large-bore needle directly from the left ventricle to the myocardium. Sen noted that Cooley had described to him, in a personal communication, Cooley's use of transmyocardial acupuncture in several desperate cases of insufficient myocardial perfusion in the 1960s [27]. Sen

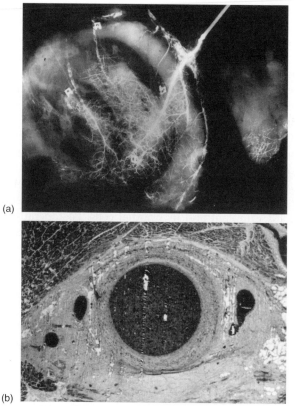

(a)

(b)

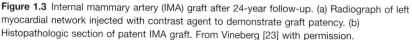

Figure 1.3 Internal mammary artery (IMA) graft after 24-year follow-up. (a) Radiograph of left myocardial network injected with contrast agent to demonstrate graft patency. (b) Histopathologic section of patent IMA graft. From Vineberg [23] with permission.

speculated that the transmyocardial channels would facilitate blood flow to the bed made more receptive of this flow by the proliferation of the microcirculation in response to chronic myocardial ischemia. Creation of this alternate route of blood flow was an attempt to duplicate the reptilian circulation (Figure 1.4). In the reptile, the coronary arteries are small, perfusing less than one-tenth of the myocardial thickness, and most of the myocardium is supplied directly from the ventricular cavity to the myocardial sinusoids during systolic contraction. This attempt by Sen to improve myocardial perfusion through direct ventriculo-myocardial communication was an early clinical application of transmyocardial revascularization (TMR) [28].

In 1967, while performing a Vineberg procedure on a 61-year-old man with triple coronary artery disease, Hershey and White [29] employed Sen's acupuncture technique as a last resort to save the patient from refractory ventricular fibrillation. After puncturing the left ventricle approximately 100 times with a 2.5-mm intravenous knobbed cannula and applying prolonged intermit-

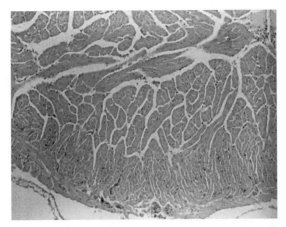

Figure 1.4 Histologic cross-section showing non-compacted myocardium of snake heart.

tent cardiac compressions, revascularization was achieved and normal ventricular rhythm was restored. This allowed the Vineberg procedure to be completed. Angiography almost a year later showed that the Vineberg implants had failed to form anastomoses with the distal coronary vessels, thus suggesting that the patient's recovery may have been due to the transmyocardial acupuncture procedure. In 2000, Hershey [30] reported that the patient remained well and angina free after 14 years of follow-up.

Shortly after Sen and Hershey published their initial reports, Pifarré *et al.* [31] raised questions about the effectiveness of myocardial revascularization by transmyocardial acupuncture. On the basis of their pressure measurements in implanted venous grafts, Pifarré *et al.* believed that no pressure gradient existed between the ventricular cavity and the myocardium. However, later studies by Nematzadeh *et al.* [32] showed not only that Pifarré's indirect pressure measurements were flawed, but also that there was a persistent positive pressure gradient between the ventricular cavity and the myocardium.

Studies at the Texas Heart Institute in Houston using a more exacting and accurate transducer-tipped catheter measurement technique showed that the intramyocardial pressure (IMP) is consistently lower than the left ventricular pressure (LVP) throughout the cardiac cycle (Figure 1.5) [33]. These pressure measurements confirming the persistent positive gradient between the ventricular cavity and myocardium confirmed that unidirectional flow to the myocardium is possible through patent myocardial pathways.

The interest in indirect myocardial revascularization subsided with the successful introduction of direct CABG in the late 1960s. The CABG procedure resulted in the restoration of coronary artery blood flow and significant improvement in the surgical treatment of coronary artery disease. However, by the late 1970s, late occlusion of venous bypass grafts was being observed with increasing frequency. If the occlusion also resulted in deterioration of the clinical status of the patient, then the more arduous and risky coronary redo surgery

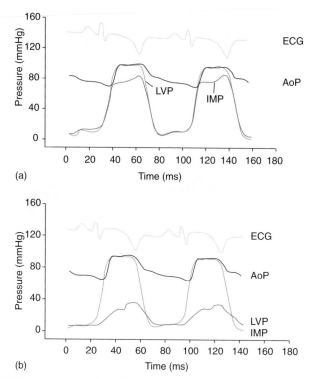

Figure 1.5 Pressure measurements made using a transducer-tipped catheter technique. Intramyocardial pressure at (a) the subendocardial level, (b) the subepicardial level. These pressure measurements demonstrate a persistent positive gradient between ventricle and myocardium and indicate the feasibility of unidirectional flow to the myocardium through patent myocardial pathways. After Frazier and Kadipasaoglu [33] with permission.

became the only alternative. This scenario renewed interest in the indirect myocardial revascularization techniques that had preceded the introduction of CABG surgery.

In 1981, Mirhoseini and Cayton [34] reported their attempt to create patent transmyocardial channels in canine hearts using a CO_2 laser (0–400 W) without producing fibrosis or scarring. In brief, they ligated the left anterior descending (LAD) coronary artery in four experimental groups of dogs and then subjected three of these groups to varying amounts of laser treatment of the myocardium. All dogs in the control group died within 20 minutes of ligation, whereas 100% survival was reported in the dogs that received laser treatment on a large area of their left ventricles perfused by the LAD. Histologic and microscopic examinations of the dogs sacrificed at 6 and 8 months after laser treatment revealed patent transmyocardial channels.

Two years later, Mirhoseini *et al.* [35] presented a clinical case report detailing the results of this laser technique as performed on a 65-year-old male with three-vessel coronary artery disease and LAD obstruction. After implanting four aortocoronary bypass grafts, this group used the CO_2 laser to create channels in the hypokinetic area of the left ventricle while the patient remained on cardiopulmonary bypass. Evaluation of postoperative technetium-99m stannous pyrophosphate (Tc-PYP) scans showed normalization of perfusion in the area of laser application.

Further experiments with TMR were performed at the Kobe University School of Medicine in Japan by Okada *et al*. [36]. In their experimental model, the researchers utilized the CO_2 laser to create myocardial channels in dogs whose hearts had been rendered ischemic. CO_2 was uniquely suitable for the creation of such channels by virtue of its ability to vaporize small 100-μm sections of the ventricle with minimal lateral injury. In 1985, after achieving promising experimental results, Okada *et al*. performed TMR as sole therapy on a 55-year-old man with severe angina and a history of pericardiectomy. As bypass was not technically possible, a CO_2 laser with an output of 85 W was used to create transmyocardial channels in the left ventricle of the patient's beating heart. The patient survived, and preoperative and postoperative assessments of cardiac catheterization data and electrocardiographic recordings did not demonstrate any abnormal changes. Okada's 12-year postoperative follow-up of the patient confirmed the success of this first reported clinical use of TMR as sole therapy [37].

Mirhoseini *et al*. [38] further assessed the safety and effectiveness of the CO_2 laser by performing TMR in conjunction with CABG on 12 patients with histories of recurrent angina pectoris. Between 10 and 12 laser channels were created in viable myocardial sites where grafting would not have been feasible. The combination therapy resulted in a 100% survival rate, reduced angina, and improved myocardial perfusion as revealed by postoperative left ventriculography and thallium stress testing.

In 1990, PLC Medical Systems, Inc. introduced the 1000-W CO_2 Heart Laser™ [39], which allowed TMR to be performed on a beating heart using a single pulse. In comparison with the 85-W laser, this high-powered laser fires one pulse in synchrony with the R wave of the electrocardiogram, at the point of maximal ventricular distention. The distention improves precision and aids in the creation of straight channels; the large amount of blood in the ventricle serves to protect the heart by absorbing the CO_2 laser emission, thereby protecting against injury to the ventricular wall opposite the channel created by the laser.

In the same year, Frazier and Cooley were approached by PLC Medical Systems, Inc. to investigate use of the CO_2 laser for treatment of angina at the Texas Heart Institute. They agreed to embark on this study only if improvement in perfusion could be demonstrated with this technology. The treatment of angina alone is beset with problems related to the placebo effect. This required a clear measurement of improved perfusion to confirm a plausible relationship between the channel creation and relief of anginal symptoms. The first TMR cases enrolled in the Texas Heart Institute study were patients with severe angina related to demonstrated impaired perfusion. These patients were not suitable candidates for surgical revascularization or interventional cardiology. The laser was applied off-pump and with consistency in regards to the laser energy applied and the number of channels created. Positron emission tomography (PET) scanning was performed to demonstrate a perfusion deficit before intervention was considered. At the time, the PET technology was the most precise scientific means of measuring myocardial perfusion. In addition, it allowed the balance between endocardial and epicardial perfusion to be measured. PET studies were performed before intervention (at baseline) and at 3 and 6 months. There was consistent clinical improvement in the angina but, more importantly, there was statistically significant improvement in endocardial perfusion (Figure 1.6). The scientist who interpreted endocardial perfusion was not involved in applying the therapy [40]. This expensive and time-consuming study provided

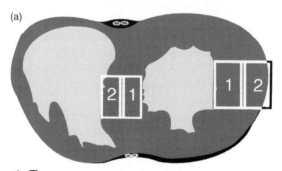

1. Tracer concentration [ ] measured in myocardial regions of interest

2. Regional perfusion ratios calculated from

$$\frac{SE_n}{SE_p} = \frac{[Region\ 1]}{[Region\ 2]}$$

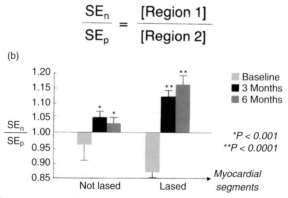

Figure 1.6 (a) Short-axis diagram of myocardium showing subendocardial (SE_n) (1) and subepicardial (SE_p) (2) regions evaluated for perfusion by positron emission tomography (PET). (b) Graph comparing regional radioactive tracer uptake myocardial perfusion in lased and non-lased myocardium during stress at baseline, 3 months, and 6 months. *P* values vs. baseline. From Frazier *et al.* [40] with permission.

convincing evidence of a relationship between improved endocardial perfusion achieved by laser therapy alone.

Between 1992 and 1995, 200 patients underwent TMR as an independent therapy in a non-randomized study at eight different medical centers in the USA [41]. In accordance with the inclusion criteria, the patients had Canadian Cardiovascular Society (CCS) class III or IV angina refractory to medical therapy, had reversible ischemia, and were not candidates for percutaneous transluminal coronary angioplasty, CABG, or cardiac transplantation. Specifically, 20% and 80% of these patients were classified as CCS class III and IV, respectively. Within 12 months after TMR, 13 patients underwent additional procedures, and three of them died as a result. At 1-year follow-up, the overall survival was 83%; postoperative evaluation at 3, 6, and 12 months demonstrated a significant decrease in the patients' CCS angina classifications and improvement of myocardial perfusion. TMR therapy was considered successful if there was a postoperative decrease of two angina classes. By this criterion, statistically significant anginal improvement was achieved. More importantly, blinded, unbiased interpretation of the myocardial perfusion studies (thallium scans) revealed a statistically significant improvement in perfusion in these patients.

A pivotal trial was initiated in 1995. This study was a prospective, multicenter, randomized trial to compare the safety and efficacy of CO_2-induced TMR versus maximal medical therapy for anginal relief [42,43]. A total of 192 patients were randomized in the study. Patients were evaluated at 3, 6, and 12 months in terms of CCS classification, quality of life, and myocardial perfusion as shown by thallium-201 single photon-emission computed tomography (SPECT) scanning. After 1 year, 72% of the TMR group showed improvement in angina symptoms (i.e., an improvement of two or more CCS classes) compared with only 13% of the medical management group (Figure 1.7) [42]. Experienced interpreters at a leading cardiovascular center who were blinded as to the mode of therapy administered assessed myocardial ischemia. Their interpretations showed a statistically significant improvement in perfusion in the TMR-treated patients and a worsening of perfusion in the patients managed medically (Figure 1.8) [42]. This study led to Food and Drug Administration (FDA) approval of the use of the CO_2 laser as sole therapy on August 20, 1998.

The unique nature of the coronary circulation has been well documented over the last 300 years. The peculiar physiologic status of the heart, which renders it incapable of extracting oxygen when faced with an oxygen debt, makes it singularly dependent on blood supply (Figure 1.9) [44]. Angiogenesis (i.e., proliferation of the microcirculation) is maximized by ischemia [45]. However, the ingress of blood to the ischemic myocardium is limited by the occlusion of epicardially based coronary arteries. As the occlusion of the coronary arteries progresses, the proliferation of the microcirculation becomes increasingly important. The known presence of direct access of blood to the ischemic myocardium is enhanced by the methodologies described here. The clinical importance of these methodologies, including their ability to provide both anginal

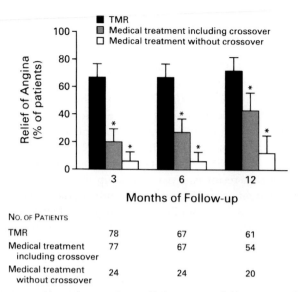

No. of Patients			
TMR	78	67	61
Medical treatment including crossover	77	67	54
Medical treatment without crossover	24	24	20

Figure 1.7 Improvement in angina symptoms with transmyocardial laser revascularization at 3, 6, and 12 months of follow-up. Angina relief was indicated by improvement of two or more Canadian Cardiovascular Society (CCS) classes. From Frazier *et al*. [42] with permission.

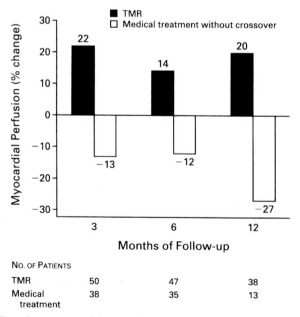

No. of Patients			
TMR	50	47	38
Medical treatment	38	35	13

Figure 1.8 Effect of transmyocardial revascularization versus medical management (MM) on left-sided myocardial perfusion. The percentage change was calculated by subtracting the number of defects reported at follow-up from the number of defect at baseline, then dividing by the number of defects at baseline. Reprinted from Frazier *et al*. [42] with permission.

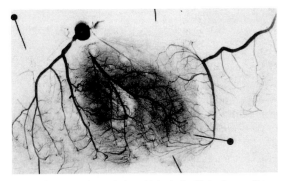

Figure 1.9 Arteriogram of postmortem pig heart injected with barium sulfate contrast dye, dissected, and unrolled. This image illustrates development of anastomoses in response to arterial occlusion by ameroid constriction. Reprinted from Schaper *et al.* [44] with permission.

relief and improved perfusion, has been demonstrated in numerous studies over the past decade. Studies with the CO_2 laser have consistently shown significant improvement in perfusion as assessed by blinded, unbiased interpretation of PET or thallium scans. A number of case reports of perfusion MRI have also demonstrated this [46,47]. TMR appears to confer a significant and consistent benefit on patients meeting the inclusion criteria of the randomized phase III trial of TMR cited above. Follow-up studies lasting up to 5 years have shown an important long-term relief of anginal symptoms in such patients [48]. Substantive improvement in patients suffering from acute myocardial infarction or advanced heart failure has not been shown to date. However, for ambulatory patients with chronic angina and preserved ventricular function, the therapeutic role of TMR has been well documented both clinically and scientifically over the last 30 years.

References

1 Vesalius A. *De humani corporis fabrica*. Basel: 1543.
2 Vieussens R. *Nouvelles découvertes sur le coeur*. Toûlouse: Jean Guillmette, 1706.
3 Raymond De Vieussens (1641–1715) French neuroanatomist and physician. *JAMA* 1968;**206**:1785–6.
4 Wearn JT. The role of the Thebesian vessels in the circulation of the heart. *J Exp Med* 1928;**47**:293–316.
5 Podolsky E. Raymond Vieussens and the affairs of the heart. *J Maine Med Assoc* 1960;**51**:362–6.
6 Wearn JT, Mettier SR, Klumpp TG, Zschiesche LJ. The nature of the vascular communications between the coronary arteries and the chambers of the heart. *Am Heart J* 1933;**9**:143–64.
7 Thebesius AC. *De circulo sanguinis in corde*. Leiden: Lugduni Batavorum, 1708.
8 Cuvier G, Duméril C. *Leçons d'anatomie comparée*. Paris: Baudouin, 1800.
9 Grant RT. An unusual anomaly of the coronary vessels in the malformed heart of a child. *Heart* 1926;**13**:273–83.

10 Stamou SC, Lefrak EA, Athari FC, Burton NA, Massimiano PS. Heart transplantation in a patient with isolated non-compaction of the left ventricular myocardium. *Ann Thorac Surg* 2004;**77**:1806–8.

11 Ivan D, Flamm SD, Abrams JA, *et al*. Isolated ventricular non-compaction in adults with idiopathic cardiomyopathy: cardiac magnetic resonance and pathologic characterization of the anomaly. *J Heart Lung Transplant* 2005;**24**:781–6.

12 Pratt FH. The nutrition of the heart through the vessels of Thebesius and the coronary veins. *Am J Physiol* 1898;**1**:86–103.

13 Leary T, Wearn JT. Two cases of complete occlusion of both coronary orifices. *J Exp Med* 1928;**47**:293.

14 Beck CS. The effect of surgical solution of chlorinated soda (Dakin's solution) in the peri-cardial cavity. *Arch Surg* 1929;**18**:1559–671.

15 Beck CS, Tichy VL, Moritz AR. Production of a collateral circulation to the heart. *Proc Soc Exp Biol Med* 1934;**32**:759–61.

16 Beck CS. A new blood supply to the heart by operation. *Surg Gynecol Obstet* 1935;**61**:407–10.

17 Beck CS, Stanton E, Batiuchok W, Leiter E. Revascularization of heart by graft of systemic artery into coronary sinus. *JAMA* 1948;**137**:436–42.

18 McAllister FF, Leighninger D, Beck CS. Revascularization by vein graft from aorta to coro-nary sinus. *Ann Surg* 1951;**133**:153–65.

19 Beck CS, Hahn RS, Leighninger DS, McAllister FF. Operation for coronary artery disease. *JAMA* 1951;**147**:1726–31.

20 Beck CS, Leighninger DS. Operations for coronary artery disease. *JAMA* 1954;**156**:1226–33.

21 Vineberg AM. Development of an anastomosis between the coronary vessels and a trans-planted internal mammary artery. *Can Med Assoc J* 1946;**55**:117–9.

22 Vineberg A. The rationale of revascularization surgery. *Dis Chest* 1969;**55**:245–9.

23 Vineberg A. Evidence that revascularization by ventricular-internal mammary artery im-plants increases longevity: twenty-four year, nine month follow-up. *J Thorac Cardiovasc Surg* 1975;**70**:381–97.

24 Goldman A, Greenstone SM, Preuss FS, Strauss SH, Chang ES. Experimental method of producing a collateral circulation into the heart directly from the left ventricle. *J Thorac Surg* 1956;**31**:364–74.

25 Massimo C, Boffi L. Myocardial revascularization by a new method of carrying blood directly from the left ventricular cavity into the coronary circulation. *J Thorac Surg* 1957;**34**:257–64.

26 Sen PK, Udwadia TE, Kinare SG, Parulkar GB. Transmyocardial acupuncture: a new ap-proach to myocardial revascularization. Proceedings of the Silver Jubilee Conference of the Association of Surgeons of India; December 1964; Bombay, India.

27 Sen PK, Daulatram J, Kinare SG, Udwadia TE, Parulkar GB. Further studies in multiple transmyocardial acupuncture as a method of myocardial revascularization. *Surgery* 1968;**64**:861–70.

28 Sen PK, Udwadia TE, Kinare SG, Parulkar GB. Transmyocardial acupuncture: a new ap-proach to myocardial revascularization. *J Thorac Cardiovasc Surg* 1965;**50**:181–9.

29 Hershey JE, White M. Transmyocardial puncture revascularization: a possible emergency adjunct to arterial implant surgery. *Geriatrics* 1969;**24**:101–8.

30 Hershey JE. Transmyocardial revascularization: could mechanical puncture be more effec-tive than puncture by laser? *Tex Heart Inst J* 2000;**27**:80–1.

31 Pifarré R, Jasuja ML, Lynch RD, Neville WE. Myocardial revascularization by transmyocar-dial acupuncture: a physiologic impossibility. *J Thoracic Cardiovasc Surg* 1969;**58**:424–31.

32 Nematzadeh D, Rose JC, Schryver T, Huang HK, Kot PA. Analysis of methodology for measurement of intramyocardial pressure. *Basic Res Cardiol* 1984;**79**:86–97.

33 Frazier OH, Kadipasaoglu KA. Transmyocardial laser revascularization. In: Buxton B, Frazier OH, Westaby S, eds. *Ischemic Heart Disease: Surgical Management*. Philadelphia: Mosby, 1999.

34 Mirhoseini M, Cayton MM. Revascularization of the heart by laser. *J Microsurg* 1981;**2**:253–60.

35 Mirhoseini M, Fisher JC, Cayton M. Myocardial revascularization by laser: a clinical report. *Lasers Surg Med* 1983;**3**:241–5.

36 Okada M, Shimizu K, Ikuta H, Horii H, Nakamura K. A new method of myocardial revascularization by laser. *Thorac Cardiovasc Surg* 1991;**39**:1–4.

37 Okada M. Transmyocardial laser revascularization (TMLR): a long way to the first successful clinical application in the world. *Ann Thorac Cardiovasc Surg* 1999;**4**:119–24.

38 Mirhoseini M, Shelgikar S, Cayton MM. New concepts in revascularization of the myocardium. *Ann Thorac Surg* 1988;**45**:415–20.

39 Crew JR. Transmyocardial revascularization by CO$_2$ laser. *Surg Tech Int* 1991;**1**:236–8.

40 Frazier OH, Cooley DA, Kadipasaoglu KA, *et al*. Myocardial revascularization with laser: preliminary findings. *Circulation* 1995;**92**(Suppl 2):58–65.

41 Horvath KA, Cohn LH, Cooley DA, *et al*. Transmyocardial laser revascularization: results of a multicenter trial with transmyocardial laser revascularization used as sole therapy for end-stage coronary artery disease. *J Thorac Cardiovasc Surg* 1997;**113**:645–54.

42 Frazier O, March R, Horvath K. Transmyocardial revascularizatin with a carbon dioxide laser in patients with end-stage coronary artery disease. *N Engl J Med* 1999;**341**:1021–8.

43 March RJ. Transmyocardial laser revascularization with the CO$_2$ laser: one year results of a randomized, controlled trial. *Semin Thorac Cardiovasc Surg* 1999;**11**:12–8.

44 Schaper W, Jageneau A, Xhonneux R. The development of collateral circulation in the pig and dog heart. *Cardiologia* 1967;**51**:321–35.

45 Schaper W. Control of coronary angiogenesis. *Eur Heart J* 1995;**16**(Suppl C):66–8.

46 Muhling OM, Wang Y, Panse P, *et al*. Transmyocardial laser revascularization preserves regional myocardial perfusion: an MRI first pass perfusion study. *Cardiovasc Res* 2003;**57**:63–70.

47 Weber C, Maas R, Steiner P, *et al*. Transmyocardial laser revascularization: the initial experiences of imaging in MRT [in German]. *Rofo Fortschr Geb Rontgenstr Neuen Bildgeb Verfahr* 1998;**169**:260–6.

48 Horvath KA, Aranki SF, Cohn LH, *et al*. Sustained angina relief 5 years after transmyocardial laser revascularization with a CO(2) laser. *Circulation* 2001;**104**(Suppl 1):81–4.

CHAPTER 2

Laser–tissue interaction

E Duco Jansen and Peter Whittaker

Introduction

The field of laser–tissue interaction has come a long way since the early days of laser, just over 4 decades ago. Proper selection of relevant primary laser para-meters such as wavelength (and, by association, depth of light penetration), pulse duration, pulse energy or laser power, repetition rate and associated para-meters such as irradiance, radiant exposure, and power density can tailor the ensuing tissue effects. This is true for all medical laser applications, including transmyocardial laser revascularization (TMR). However, 40 years after Sen *et al.* [1] first reported the creation of transmural needle puncture tracts, nearly 25 years after Mirosheini and Cayton [2] first reported the use of a laser to drill transmyocardial channels, and after over 10 000 patients worldwide have undergone TMR, the question of what type of tissue effect is desirable in TMR remains elusive. The physical mechanisms of tissue ablation with the most fre-quently used TMR lasers for TMR – the carbon dioxide laser, the holmium:YAG and the XeCl excimer lasers – is well known but the ensuing biologic effect re-sponsible for the efficacy of TMR remains largely undefined as few comparative studies have been carried out [3–5]. Several mechanisms have been hypothe-sized, ranging from placebo-like effect to laser injury-induced changes in mechanical compliance of the myocardium [6–10], and from laser-induced triggering of angiogenesis to a laser-induced denervation of the myocardium [11–13]. For many of these hypotheses, reports have been published that arrive at conclusions that are in exact opposition to others. Published reports have reached antithetic conclusions. Thus far, much of the disagreement between various studies can be attributed to the lack of consistent and appropriate animal models that accurately simulate the compromised, ischemic, diseased human myocardium. Although stimulation of angiogenesis appears to be a leading candidate hypothesis regardless of the laser used, no conclusive evi-dence has been presented to show whether the beneficial effects of the proce-dure stem from the channels created or from subsidiary adaptation elicited by other components of the laser-induced insult [14]. Add to that the wide variety of endpoints and metrics used in various studies and it is easy to see how it is difficult to arrive at any firm conclusions regarding the mechanisms of TMR.

In this chapter, a basic overview of the fundamental biophysics underlying the interaction of (laser) light with biologic tissue in the context of TMR is provided. Because terminology in this field is often ambiguous and confusing, we strive to use the nomenclature and conventions as proposed by Welch and van Gemert [15].

Conventional wisdom in the field of laser tissue interaction suggests that the holy grail in laser ablation is to remove the target material (in the case of TMR, the channel) while minimizing collateral damage to the tissue left behind. This damage can consist of thermal damage (coagulation) typically associated with longer pulse durations or of mechanical damage associated with laser-induced pressure transients or cavitation effects resulting from the explosive nature of the ablation process [16]. This mechanical damage is associated with short laser pulses. In the case of TMR, the desired reduction in collateral damage may not be so straightforward, as many studies have suggested that some damage to the remaining myocardium may in fact be a desirable feature and perhaps crucial in the efficacy of the treatment. In this chapter, predictions as to what type of mechanism is desirable or what level or kind of tissue damage should be strived for will be largely avoided because they can be speculative at best. More specific correlations to *in vivo* TMR outcomes both in animal models and in human studies can be found in Chapter 3 but even there it will be evident that, owing to an array of complexities, drawing any conclusions regarding the mechanisms of TMR is nearly impossible.

When applying laser light to biologic tissue a variety of complex interactions may occur. A comprehensive discussion of all aspects of laser–tissue interaction is clearly beyond the scope of this chapter so we limit our discussion to the most important concepts in the context of TMR. Specific tissue characteristics as well as laser parameters contribute to this diversity. Most important among tissue optical properties are the refractive index and the wavelength dependent coefficients of absorption and scattering. Together they determine the distribution of light in tissue at a certain wavelength. On the other hand, the following parameters are given by the laser radiation itself: wavelength, exposure time, laser power, applied energy, spot size, radiant exposure (energy/unit area), and irradiance (power/unit area). Of these, the wavelength and exposure time are the crucial parameters when selecting the type of interaction (Fig. 2.1).

Tissue optics

In describing the optical properties and light propagation in tissues, light is treated as photons. The primary reason for this approach is that biologic tissue is an inhomogeneous mix of compounds, many with unknown properties, at unknown and varying quantities and distributed in a variable and largely unknown fashion. Hence, analytical solutions to Maxwell's equations in this medium pose an intractable mathematical problem. The representation of light as photons presents the opportunity to apply probabilistic approaches that lend themselves particularly well to numerical solutions that are tractable in computer simulations. Photons in a turbid medium such as tissue can move randomly in all directions and may be scattered (described by its scattering

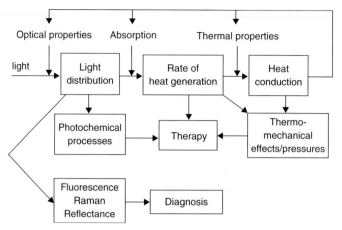

Figure 2.1 Schematic of laser–tissue interactions.

coefficient μ_s [m^{-1}]) or absorbed (described by its absorption coefficient μ_a [m^{-1}]). These coefficients, along with anisotropy, g (i.e. the direction in which a photon is scattered) and index of refraction, n, are referred to as the optical properties of a material and collectively they determine how light is distributed in tissue. When photons impinge on tissue several things can happen:

1 Some photons reflect off the surface of the material (similar to what happens to glass and other materials – Fresnel's equations also hold for tissue)

2 The majority of the photons enter the tissue, upon which the following can happen:

   (a) The photon is absorbed (and can be converted to heat, trigger a chemical reaction, or cause fluorescence emission)

   (b) The photon is scattered (bumps into a particle and changes direction but continues to exist with the same energy or wavelength). Note that scattered photons may eventually be absorbed somewhere in the tissue.

Absorption

We first consider the case when light is only absorbed. In tissue optics, absorption of photons is a crucial event; absorption is the primary event that allows a laser or other light source to cause a potentially therapeutic (or damaging) effect on a tissue. Without absorption, there is no energy transfer to the tissue and the tissue is left unaffected by the light. Molecules that absorb light are called *chromophores*. Depending on the wavelength of the laser light, different chromophores are primarily responsible for absorption of the laser radiation. These include water, blood (hemoglobin), melanin, amino acids, proteins, and fatty acids [16–18].

• *In the UV:* tissue absorption is high because of protein, amino acid, fatty acid, and DNA absorption.

• *In the visible:* whole blood (hemoglobin) is a strong absorber for some wavelengths (blue/green) but its effect is limited because the fraction of blood in tissue is small, unless one considers highly perfused tissues or the vasculature itself. Melanin is a strong absorber, again providing a small fraction of tissue on average except when considering areas with strong pigmentation such as the skin or retina.

• *In the infrared:* tissue absorption is dominated by water absorption and can vary from low (i.e., at near infrared wavelengths such as the 1064 nm Nd:YAG wavelength) to extremely high (i.e., at the water absorption peak at 2940 nm as emitted by the Er:YAG laser).

Assuming that the probability of a photon getting absorbed is much larger than the probability of that photon being scattered, we can neglect scattering. In this case the light distribution in the tissue is given by the well-known Beer's law and shows an exponential decay with depth:

$$E(z) = E_0 e^{-\mu_a(\lambda)z} \tag{1}$$

where E_0 is the irradiance (W/cm^2) in case of continuous wave lasers or radiant exposure (better known as fluence) (J/cm^2) for pulse lasers (in which case often the symbol H_0 is used). The absorption coefficient, $M_a(\lambda)$ (in units of m^{-1}) is defined as the probability that a photon is absorbed when traveling some distance Δz (i.e., $1/\mu_a$ is the mean free path a photon travels before an absorption event takes place) [15].

A related and useful parameter is the penetration depth, δ, defined as the depth in the medium at which the energy or irradiance is reduced to $1/e$ times (~37%) the incident irradiance at the surface. Per definition the penetration depth equals $1/\mu_a$ in cases where there is no scattering.

For efficient ablation, it is desirable to have a high absorption coefficient or small optical penetration depth. This results in laser energy being absorbed in a relatively shallow layer of tissue, thus rapidly heating up the small irradiated volume with relatively little energy while minimizing both the direct deposition of heat as well as thermal diffusion to surrounding tissues. In general, light in the red and near infrared part of the spectrum (600–1600 nm) is not highly absorbed. The two desired spectral windows for efficient ablation, where absorption is high, can be found below 350 nm (dominated by absorption by proteins, amino acids, and fatty acids) and above 2 μm (where water is the abundantly present chromophore). This fact is largely responsible for the selection of laser wavelengths used in TMR; the carbon dioxide laser (far infrared, $\lambda = 10.6$ μm, $\delta = 12$ μm), the holmium:YAG laser (mid-infrared, $\lambda = 2.12$ μm, $\delta = 330$ μm), and the XeCl excimer laser (UV, $\lambda = 308$ nm, $\delta = 60$ μm) all are strongly absorbed in the myocardium. Other highly absorbed wavelength such as the Er:YAG laser (mid-infrared, $\lambda = 2.94$ μm, $\delta = 1$ μm) or even other excimer lasers such as the ArF (UV, $\lambda = 193$ nm, $\delta < 1$ μm) would in principle be good candidates but suffer from issues such as limited potential of fiberoptic delivery (both the Er:YAG and the ArF), potential of inducing mutagenic effects in biologic material (ArF), and inherently low ablation rates owing to limitations in the pulse energy/laser power associated with these lasers.

Following the distribution of laser light as determined by the optical properties, the optical energy is absorbed in the tissue and in most cases converted to heat. The rate of heat generation, S, is defined as the number of photons absorbed per unit time, per unit volume (W/m^3). Mathematically, the rate of heat generation, $S(r,z)$, for every point in the tissue is expressed as the product of fluence rate, φ (the amount of light energy traveling through that point per unit time) and the probability of absorption of that light at that point. This can be written for a radially symmetrical situation as:

$$S(r,z) = \mu_a(r,z)\,\phi(r,z) \tag{2}$$

However, for the absorption dominated situation, the term φ (r,z) can be replaced by E (r,z) from equation (1). It is important to note that this is valid for continuous as well as pulsed lasers. Multiplying the rate of heat generation, S, by the total exposure time (pulse duration) gives the energy density (J/cm^3) at any point in the tissue for which the symbol, W, is used. Knowing the energy density, the temperature rise in the tissue at any point can be calculated in first approximation by:

$$\Delta T(r,z) = \frac{W(r,z)}{\rho c} \tag{3}$$

where ρ is the density (kg/m^3) and c is the specific heat ($J/kg\,K$) of the tissue. However, this approximation is valid only when heat diffusion is ignored. The validity of this assumption is debatable and is certainly not accurate when relatively long exposure times are used (relative to the thermal diffusion time).

Scattering

Given the dominance of absorption, the role of scattering can safely be ignored for these lasers (note that this is not the case when other lasers such as the Nd:YAG or near infrared diode laser are used). Hence, the discussion of scattering will be limited here. Scattering of light occurs in media that contains spatial fluctuations in the refractive index n, whether such fluctuations are discrete particles or more continuous variations in n. The scattering coefficient, μ_s (m^{-1}), is defined as the probability that a photon is absorbed when traveling some distance Δz. The mean free path of scattering is $1/\mu_s$ [15].

Light–tissue interactions

During the first decades after invention of the laser by Maiman in 1960, many studies have investigated potential interaction effects by using all types of laser systems and tissue targets. Although the number of possible combinations for the experimental parameters is unlimited, generally three different types of interaction mechanisms are classified today: photochemical, photothermal, and photomechanical [19]. Each of these interaction mechanisms is discussed in detail in this chapter and the physical principles governing these interactions are reviewed.

Before going into detail, an interesting observation deserves to be stated. All these seemingly different interaction types share a common property: the characteristic radiant exposure [J/cm^2] ranges from approximately $1 J/cm^2$ to $1000 J/cm^2$. This is surprising because the irradiance itself varies by more than 15 orders of magnitude. Thus, a single parameter distinguishes and primarily controls these processes: the duration of the laser exposure which is largely similar to the interaction time itself [20]. With regards to TMR, the typical exposure times or pulse durations associated with the candidate TMR lasers span nearly 6 orders of magnitude and range from approximately 100 ns (for the XeCl laser) to 250 μs (for the holmium:YAG laser). It should be noted that these pulse durations are dictated by device characteristics rather than being based on any sort of rational design aimed at optimizing clinical outcome. For the carbon dioxide laser, which technically is a continuous wave rather than a pulsed laser, the typical exposure time is 40–50 ms. Associated with this difference in pulse duration is the fact that both the holmium and excimer lasers require multiple pulses to traverse the myocardium while the carbon dioxide laser crates a channel in one single shot. It should also be noted that although the exposure time of the carbon dioxide laser is 40 ms, the true interaction time within a zone equal to the penetration depth is approximately 24 μs because the ablation front moves at a significant speed of 500 mm/s.

A log–log plot of irradiance versus pulse duration with the basic interaction mechanisms is show in Figure 2.2. In this figure the photomechanical mechanisms are separated in three subcategories: photo-ablation, plasma-induced ablation, and photodisruption. In the graphs the two diagonals show constant radiant exposures at $1 J/cm^2$ and $1000 J/cm^2$, respectively. According to this graph, the timescale can roughly be divided in three major sections: continuous wave or exposure times >1 s for photochemical interactions, 100 s down to 1 μs for photothermal interactions, and 1 μs and shorter for photomechanical inter-

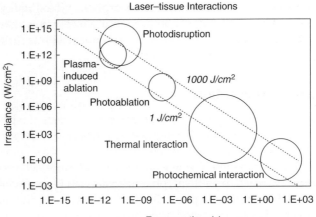

Figure 2.2 Laser–tissue interaction regimes. Note that despite the fact that the irradiance varies over more than 15 orders of magnitude, the characteristic radiant exposure (J/cm^2) ranges from approximately $1 J/cm^2$ to $1000 J/cm^2$. Figure adapted from Niemz [20].

actions. It should be clear, however, that these boundaries are not strict and adjacent interaction types cannot always be separated. Thus, overlap in these main regions does exist. For example, in the range of 1 μs to several hundreds of μs, the interaction mechanisms typically have photothermal as well as photomechanical components to them, while many photochemical interactions also exhibit photothermal components. Finally, there is the possibility that multiple pulses of a particular interaction type collectively contribute to another interaction type. For example, even pulses of a duration of 100 ps, each of which have negligible thermal interactions, may add up to a measurable temperature increase if applied at repetition rates of 20 Hz or higher, depending on the laser. We now consider each of the main interaction mechanisms in some more detail.

Photochemical interactions

We will only briefly discuss photochemical interactions (for an excellent overview of mechanisms and some applications see chapter 3 of Niemz' book *Laser–Tissue Interaction* [20]). In brief, the group of photochemical interactions is based on the fact that light can induce chemical effects and reactions within macromolecules or tissues. The most obvious example of this is created by nature itself: photosynthesis. In the field of medical laser applications, photochemical interaction mechanisms have a role during photodynamic therapy (PDT) [21]. Frequently, biostimulation is also attributed to photochemical interactions, although this is not scientifically established.

Photochemical interactions take place at very low irradiances (typically 1 W/cm^2) and long exposure times ranging from seconds to tens of minutes. Careful selection of laser parameters (most notably wavelength) yields a radiation distribution inside the tissue that is primarily determined by scattering. In most cases, wavelengths in the red and near infrared part of the spectrum (600–900 nm) are used because of their low absorption and resulting deep penetration in tissue. Because the role of photochemical effects in the context of TMR is thought to be essentially non-existent, we will not elaborate further on this mechanism.

Photothermal interactions

Photothermal interactions include a large group of interaction types resulting from the transformation of absorbed light energy to heat, leading to a local temperature increase. Thermal effects can be induced by either continuous wave (CW) or pulsed laser radiation. While photochemical processes are often governed by a specific reaction pathway, photothermal effects generally tend to be non-specific and are mediated primarily by absorption of optical energy and secondly governed by fundamental principles of heat transport. Depending on the duration and peak value of the temperature achieved, different effects such as coagulation, vaporization, melting, or carbonization may be distinguished. An excellent overview of these interaction regimes can be found in Thomsen

[22]. It is essential to emphasize that thermal interactions in tissue are typically governed by rate processes (i.e. not just the temperature has a role but the duration for which the tissue is exposed to a particular temperature is also a parameter of major importance).

Once deposited in tissue and given sufficient time, the traditional mechanism of heat transfer applies to laser-irradiated biologic tissues. Heat flows in biologic tissue whenever a temperature difference exists. The transfer of thermal energy is governed by the laws of thermodynamics:

1 energy is conserved; and

2 heat flows from areas of high temperature to areas of low temperature.

The primary mechanisms of heat transfer to consider are conduction, convection, and radiation [23]. In addition, metabolic heat, perfusion, and evaporation can have important effects on the overall temperature field of the laser-irradiated tissue.

Ablation

The word ablation comes from the Latin "ablatus" which means "to remove." There are two types of meaning of the word ablation. In a physics/engineering sense it refers to the physical removal of material (tissue), while in the medical/biologic sense it refers to the physiologic removal of tissue (i.e., causing the tissue to stop performing the processes needed for survival and/or function of the tissue, that is killing the cells but not necessarily physically removing them).

Generally, below the boiling point of water, thermal interactions are dominated by protein denaturation and tissue coagulation, resulting in many cases in cell apoptosis or necrosis. Several medical applications use this type of interaction to achieve the clinical endpoint. For example, during interstitial hyperthermia, relatively weakly absorbed wavelengths are used combined with long exposure times (minutes) to slowly coagulate or cook a mass of tissue such as a tumor using fiberoptic delivery of laser light.

Above 100°C, the thermal interactions become dominated by evaporation of water and we typically operate in the regime where physical material removal occurs. In this case the goal is usually to remove or ablate the target tissue while minimizing the damage to the tissue left behind. Some notable exceptions to this paradigm include those applications where, in addition to cutting with the laser, some coagulation is desirable, for instance when the target tissue is highly vascularized. The desired endpoint in this regard during TMR is still unknown. The amount of collateral thermal damage is largely determined by the amount of heat that can diffuse out of the irradiated tissue prior to the ejection of this material. Hence, it will be intuitive that the pulse duration is a critical parameter.

Continuous wave ablation

The clinically used carbon dioxide laser (TMR) is a continuous wave laser. Parameters of importance for this type of laser are power (energy/unit time), irradiance (power/unit area), and the duration of the laser exposure (time that the laser is emitting radiation). The chronology of the events that occur during continuous wave ablation of soft tissue has been well documented [24–26] and generally follows the following sequence. Upon absorption of laser energy by tissue water, rapid heating occurs. As energy is spent on vaporization (latent heat), the temperature ranges from 100 to 150°C. After local desiccation of tissue, the temperature continues to rise to approximately 350–450°C, at which point carbonization and ablation (tissue removal) takes place, thus exposing new cooler layers below. This process continues as the ablation front moves deeper into the tissue with a fairly constant velocity. Although the CO_2 laser has been used in many medical applications since the early days of laser medicine, thus far treatment has involved lasers of typically no more than 80 W. TMR represents the first clinical application of a high-power, continuous wave CO_2 laser (800 W), similar to those used in material processing (large-scale cutting and welding of metals). By increasing the power to these levels, the ablation front will move so rapidly into the tissue that thermal diffusion to surrounding tissue may be reduced. An added advantage is that by increasing the laser power, the time needed to create a transmural channel is reduced. This in turn enables drilling of the entire channel with a single burst of energy during diastole.

Based on the very nature of the interaction of laser radiation with tissue, the damage mechanisms may be thermal or mechanical [19,22]. In brief, mechanical damage is caused by subsurface explosion of heated tissue material (in particular in cases where the absorption coefficient is relatively small), while thermal damage is caused by two sources:

1 direct deposition of heat in layers beyond the point where the energy density was sufficient for ablation (i.e., below threshold); and

2 thermal diffusion (from heated tissue to surrounding cooler tissue).

With regards to the latter, if the laser pulse is longer than the thermal diffusion time (i.e., the time it takes for heat to diffuse out of the irradiated volume), the thermal energy propagates into the surrounding tissue during the laser pulse, causing denaturation, coagulation, and significant thermal damage to adjacent tissues. The irony is that reducing the pulse duration in order to minimize the amount of heat diffusion that can take place before heated material is ejected will cause the ablation process to be even more explosive and violent, thus increasing the collateral mechanical damage to the tissue.

Pulsed laser ablation

The rationale of using pulsed lasers instead of CW lasers is largely attributable to the desire to reduce the extent of the zone of thermal damage. Using highly absorbed infrared lasers (i.e., the holmium:YAG) the ablation process is largely a process of water vaporization and photothermal disruption of tissue. This process is similar to ablation with CW irradiation and is associated with rapid subsurface pressure build-up with possible superheating. Eventually, an explosion occurs which may be accompanied by an acoustic transient or shock wave and rapid ejection of tissue fragments. The influence of the laser parameters on the ablation process, temperature and pressure associated with the vapor bubble formation, and the interaction between the vapor bubble formation and tissue mechanical properties have been well documented. For the XeCl excimer laser the ablation mechanism is only slightly more complicated. The mechanism of interaction of this laser (λ = 308 nm) is different from the ArF excimer laser (λ = 193 nm), which is the laser that is widely used for LASIK procedures. Whereas the photons from the ArF laser have sufficient energy to directly break molecular bonds, the photons from the XeCl laser do not. Hence, the role of so-called "cold ablation" based on direct photochemistry is negligible with the XeCl excimer laser [27,28]. Instead, the mechanism is predominantly photothermal and hence similar to that described for the infrared lasers. Indeed, such a photothermal mechanism is supported by documented temperature rises of more than 70°C during XeCl laser ablation [29,30]. The dominant chromophores at this wavelength include proteins, amino acids, and fatty acids. Subsequent to absorption by these chromophores, the thermal energy is almost instantaneously transferred to the abundantly present tissue water molecules. From this point on, the ablation process is in essence identical to the infrared process in that a rapidly expanding and collapsing vapor bubble is formed which is capable of significant tissue tearing and which may be accompanied by a pressure or shock wave. Thus, the major differences between the UV XeCl excimer laser and the mid-infrared lasers such as the holmium:YAG, besides the microscopic site of absorption, are the penetration depth of the laser light and the inherent and device-specific pulse duration generated by the laser. Clearly, these will have an effect on related parameters such as the ablation threshold and ablation efficiency. Nevertheless, the XeCl is a potential candidate laser for TMR [31]. For a more detailed discussion of the physics of pulsed laser ablation of tissue, we refer the reader to a superb and comprehensive overview published by Vogel and Venugopalan [32].

Photomechanical interaction

Photomechanical interaction includes mechanisms associated with photoablation, explosive vaporization, plasma-induced ablation, and laser-induced acoustic (shock waves). Note that even though we discuss them separately, photothermal and photomechanical events are closely intertwined. In the context of the ablation process, we have already discussed the explosive vaporization process. While tissue rupture by explosive vaporization is mechanical in nature, it is thermal in origin. In the context of TMR, explosive vaporization, bubble formation and, secondary to that, tissue rupture and even forced convection have a major role in determining the zone of damage surrounding the transmural channels. In addition to these mechanisms, the formation of laser-induced acoustic transients or shock waves can result in sometimes subtle types of tissue damage. While a careful and detailed analysis of laser-induced acoustic phenomena is beyond the scope of this chapter, a brief overview of the main concepts may be important because part of the mechanical damage to tissue, especially in the case of very short laser pulses (i.e., <1 μs), may be caused by these laser-induced pressure waves.

In absorbing samples, three mechanisms of pressure wave generation can be identified [33]:

1 thermoelastic effect;

2 ablative recoil stress; and

3 collapse pressure generated upon collapse of the rapidly expanding and subsequently collapsing vapor bubble.

All materials expand upon heating as an increase in temperature results in a larger equilibrium atomic spacing. This expansion is driven by internal forces and if hindered, as in the case of a constrained body or by the material inertia under conditions of rapid heating, large stresses develop. This is known as the thermoelastic effect. For the thermoelastic pressures to be of importance, the laser pulse must be shorter than the stress confinement time (i.e., the time it takes for the pressure increase to diffuse out of the irradiated volume). Practically speaking, for the highly absorbed wavelengths used in TMR the laser pulses used are not sufficiently short to allow pressure build-up and hence this effect is unlikely to play a major role.

The second source of pressure wave generation is attributed to the ablative removal of material from a tissue surface. Regardless of whether or not conditions of stress confinement are met (and hence thermoelastic expansion induced pressure waves are created), short laser pulses when containing sufficient energy can cause the explosive phase change of water. This explosive surface vaporization or phase explosion results in the forceful ejection of debris. In turn, the conservation of momentum dictates that the force of the ejected debris must be compensated by an equal force in the opposite direction. The net result is that if explosive ablation occurs, a second source of pressure wave generation – the ablative recoil force – causes forceful compressive stress waves into the tissue. The amplitude of these pressure waves scales with the laser radiant exposure.

Regardless of their origin, laser-induced stress waves can contribute to the ablation mechanism and may inflict tissue damage, even far away from the irradiated zone. As the generated stress wave travels through the tissue at the speed of sound (in the case of an acoustic transient) or at supersonic velocities (in the case of a shock wave), the local pressure transiently increases and decreases. It is likely that these transients affect cellular membranes and subcellular structures.

Plasma-induced ablation

A last regime of laser–tissue interactions involves the use of ultrashort (ps and fs) pulse lasers. Using these types of lasers, the peak irradiances are so high ($>10^{12}$ W/cm^2) that the electric field of the light permeating the medium is capable of ionizing the material, a process known as plasma formation or dielectric breakdown. This can occur even when the linear absorption of the wavelengths used is negligible. The result is the generation of a small cloud of free electrons and positively charged ions, known as a plasma. Once formed the plasma becomes self-absorbing, causing the remaining laser energy to be efficiently coupled in the growing plasma. Prerequisite for the occurrence of a plasma is:

1 a very short laser pulse (in order to increase the power, even when only small pulse energies are used); and

2 a small spot size (the irradiance scales with the inverse of the spot radius squared).

The resulting plasma typically involves small volumes (several microns) but this microscopic volume may reach local temperatures exceeding thousands of degrees. In the moments immediately following the laser pulse, the plasma energy diffuses to the surrounding tissue (water). The result is virtually always the formation of a pressure or shock wave and the rapid vaporization of tissue water, resulting in an explosive ablation process. Notable medical applications of this technology include the use of Q-switched Nd:YAG lasers (few ns, 1064 nm) in cataract surgery and, more recently, the use of an fs laser for the creation of bladeless corneal flaps in LASIK surgery [34]. In the latter case, the near infrared laser is focused inside the corneal stroma at the desired depth and each fs pulse generates a rapidly expanding and collapsing microbubble of approximately 3 μm in diameter which separates corneal layers. The laser beam is scanned over the cornea at 20 kHz and adjacent voids together create a clean hinged flap. Other exciting applications of plasma-induced microevents have been reported in cellular manipulation and subcellular microsurgery [35]. Initial reports of the use of this type of laser–tissue interaction for TMR have appeared in recent years [36]. While ablation can be achieved with virtually no collateral damage in this fashion, it is unclear if this is desirable in the context of TMR. A detailed discussion of the physics of laser-induced plasma formation and photodisruption is beyond the scope of this chapter and the reader is referred to Niemz [20].

Biologic effects

Regardless of the source of damage (thermal, mechanical, or even photochemical), biologic tissue typically responds to lethal damage with either a necrotic or apoptotic response. The exact decision of whether a cell will move down the necrotic or apoptotic pathway in response to laser-induced damage is largely unknown. Some evidence exists that oxidative stress, as generated for example in photodynamic therapy, shows a marked upregulation of apoptotic markers [37]. Similar, sublethal damage has been shown to upregulate the expression of molecular chaperones such as the heat shock protein family, in particular hsp70 [38,39]. In many lethal thermal damage scenarios, the biologic response can be classified as a coagulation necrosis, followed by a normal wound healing response which includes formation of granulation tissue, scar formation, and scar remodeling [40]. The role of any of these processes in the TMR-treated myocardium is still largely unknown.

Conclusions

In summary, lasers are capable of producing channels in the myocardium. Understanding the interaction of laser radiation with tissue, in particular the role of wavelength, pulse duration, and pulse energy or power, allows the channel and collateral damage to be tailor-made. Long pulses cause collateral thermal damage to tissue adjacent to the ablation crater while short pulses cause collateral mechanical damage. Thermal damage can be the result of thermal diffusion or direct irradiation of tissue at subthreshold levels. Mechanical damage can be the result of explosive vaporization or laser-induced pressure transients. The latter can originate by thermoelastic expansion, ablative recoil, or as a side-effect of rapid explosive vaporization. To a large extent, however, the relevant laser parameters are dictated by the specific physical properties of the various lasers used and the capabilities of delivery systems rather than by any sort of optimization process of the clinical procedure. In order to achieve efficient ablation, wavelengths that are highly absorbed by soft tissue are candidates for TMR. This includes the carbon dioxide, holmium:YAG, and XeCl excimer lasers. Of these, all but the carbon dioxide laser can be fiber delivered and hence are potential candidates for non-invasive approaches such as percutaneous myocardial revascularization (PMR). Ultimately, what is missing is even a rudimentary understanding of the biologic response of the myocardium to the channel formation and collateral damage incurred during TMR procedure. Until such understanding is achieved it is difficult, if not impossible, to specify optimal laser parameters that could achieve optimal success in transmyocardial revascularization.

References

1 Sen PK, Udwadia TE, Kinare SG, Parulkar GB. Transmyocardial revascularization: a new approach to myocardial revascularization. *J Thorac Cardiovasc Surg* 1965;**50**:181–9.

2 Mirhoseini M, Cayton MM. Revascularization of the heart by laser. *J Microsurg* 1981;**2**:253–60.

3 Kadipasaoglu KA, Frazier OH. Transmyocardial laser revascularization: effect of laser parameters on tissue ablation and cardiac perfusion. *Semin Thorac Cardiovasc Surg* 1999;**11**:4–11.

4 Hartman RA, Whittaker P. The physics of transmyocardial revascularization. *J Clin Laser Med Surg* 1997;**15**:255–9.

5 Kadipasaoglu KA, Sartori M, Masai T, *et al.* Interoperative arrhythmias and tissue damage during transmyocardial laser revascularization. *Ann Thorac Surg* 1999;**67**:423–31.

6 Gassler N, Rastar R, Hentz MW. Angiogenesis and expression of tenascin after transmural revascularization. *Histol Histopathol* 1999;**14**:81–7.

7 Roethy W, Yamamoto N, Burkhoff D. An examination of potential mechanisms underlying transmyocardial laser revascularization induced increases in myocardial blood flow. *Semin Thorac Cardiovasc Surg* 1999;**11**:24–8.

8 Hughes GC, Lowe JE, Kypson AP, *et al.* Neovascularization after transmyocardial laser revascularization in a model of chronic ischemia. *Ann Thorac Surg* 1998;**66**:2029–36.

9   Malekan R, Reynolds C, Narula N, *et al*. Angiogenesis in transmyocardial laser revascular-
    ization: a non-specific response to injury. *Circulation* 1998;**19**(Suppl 2):62–5.

10 Pelletier MP, Giaid A, Sivaraman A, *et al*. Angiogenesis and growth factor expression in a
    model of transmyocardial revascularization. *Ann Thorac Surg* 1998;**66**:12–8.

11 Hirsch GM, Thompson GW, Arora RC, *et al*. Transmyocardial laser revascularization does
    not denervate the canine heart. *Ann Thorac Surg* 1999;**68**:468–9.

12 Kwong KF, Schuessler RB, Kanellopoulos GK, *et al*. Nontransmural laser treatment incom-
    pletely denervates canine myocardium. *Circulation* 1998;**19**(Suppl 2):67–71.

13 Al-Sheikh T, Allen KB, Straka SP, *et al*. Cardiac sympathetic denervation after transmyocar-
    dial laser revascularization. *Circulation* 1999;**100**:135–40.

14 Domkowski PW, Biswas SS, Steenbergen C, *et al*. Histological evidence of angiogenesis 9
    months after transmyocardial laser revascularization. *Circulation* 2001;**103**:469–71.

15 Welch AJ, van Gemert MJC. *Optical Thermal Response of Laser-Irradiated Tissue*. Plenum Press,
    1995.

16 Jansen ED. Laser tissue interaction. In: Wnek GE, Bowlin GL, eds. *Encyclopedia of Biomateri-
    als and Biomedical Engineering*, 1st edn. New York, NY: Marcel Dekker, 2004: 883–91.

17 Cheong WF, Prahl SA, Welch AJ. A review of the optical properties of biological tissue. *IEEE
    Trans Quantum Elect* 1990;**26**:2166–85.

18 Hale GM, Querry MR. Optical constants of water in the 200 nm to 200 mm wavelength re-
    gion. *Appl Optics* 1973;**12**:555–63.

19 Jacques SL. Laser–tissue interactions: photochemical, photothermal and photomechanical.
    Surg Clin North Am 1992;**72**:531–58.

20 Niemz M. *Laser–Tissue Interaction*. Berlin: Springer-Verlag, 1996.

21 Ochsner M. Photophysical and photobiological processes in the photodynamic therapy of
    tumours. *J Photochem Photobiol B* 2000;**39**:1–18.

22 Thomsen SL. Pathologic analysis of photothermal and photomechanical effects of laser–tis-
    sue interactions. *Photochem Photobiol* 1991;**53**:825–35.

23 Incropera FP, DeWitt DP. *Introduction to Conduction*. New York, NY: John Wiley & Sons,
    1990.

24 LeCarpentier GL, Motamedi M, McMath LP, *et al*. Continuous wave laser ablation of tissue:
    analysis of thermal and mechanical events. *IEEE Trans Biomed Eng* 1993;**40**:188–200.

25 Verdaasdonk RM, Borst C, van Gemert MJC. Explosive onset of continuous wave tissue ab-
    lation. *Phys Med Biol* 1990;**35**:1129–44.

26 Jansen ED, Frenz M, Kadipasaoglu KA, *et al*. Laser–tissue interaction during transmyocar-
    dial laser revascularization. *Ann Thorac Surg* 1997;**63**:640–7.

27 Oraevsky AA, Jacques SL, Pettit GH, *et al*. XeCl ablation of atherosclerotic aorta: optical
    properties and energy pathways. *Lasers Surg Med* 1992;**12**:585–97.

28 Clarke RH, Isner JM, Donaldson RF, *et al*. Gas chromatographic-light microscopic correla-
    tive analysis of excimer laser photoablation of cardiovascular tissues: evidence for a ther-
    mal mechanism. *Circ Res* 1987;**60**:429–37.

29 Jansen ED, Le TH, Welch AJ. Excimer, Ho:YAG and Q-switched Ho:YAG ablation of aorta: a
    comparison of temperatures and tissue damage *in vitro*. *Appl Opt* 1993;**32**:526–34.

30 Gijsbers GHM, Sprangers RLH, Keijzer M, *et al*. Some laser-tissue interactions in 308 nm ex-
    cimer laser coronary angioplasty. *J Interv Cardiol* 1990;**3**:231–41.

31 Shehada RE, Papaioannou T, Mansour HN, *et al*. Excimer laser (308 nm) based transmy-
    ocardial laser revascularization: effects of the lasing parameters on myocardial histology.
    Lasers Surg Med 2001;**29**:85–91.

32 Vogel A, Venugopalan V. Mechanisms of pulsed laser ablation of biological tissues. *Chem
    Rev* 2003;**130**:577–644.

33 Esenaliev RO, Oraevsky AA, Letokhov VS, Karabutov AA, Malinsky TV. Studies of acoustical and shock waves in the pulsed laser ablation of biotissue. *Lasers Surg Med* 1993;**13**:470–84.

34 Ratkay-Traub I, Ferincz IE, Juhasz T, Kurtz RM, Krueger RR. First clinical results with the femtosecond neodynium-glass laser in refractive surgery. *J Refract Surg* 2003;**19**:94–103.

35 Venugopalan V, Guerra A 3rd, Nahen K, Vogel A. Role of laser-induced plasma formation in pulsed cellular microsurgery and micromanipulation. *Phys Rev Lett* 2002;**88**:078103.

36 Ogura M, Sato S, Ishihara M, *et al*. Myocardium tissue ablation with high-peak-power nanosecond 1,064- and 532-nm pulsed lasers: influence of laser-induced plasma. *Lasers Surg Med* 2002;**31**:136–141.

37 Oleinick NL, Morris RL, Belichenko I. The role of apoptosis in response to photodynamic therapy: what, where, why, and how. *Photochem Photobiol Sci* 2003;**1**:1–21.

38 Beckham JT, Mackanos MA, Crooke C, *et al*. Assessment of cellular response to thermal laser injury through bioluminescence imaging of hsp70. *Photochem Photobiol* 2004;**79**:76–85.

39 Desmettre T, Maurage CA, Mordon S. Heat shock protein hyperexpression on chorioretinal layers after transpupillary thermotherapy. *Invest Ophthalmol Vis Sci* 2001;**42**:2976–80.

40 Wu NJ, Jansen ED, Davidson JM. Comparison of MMP-13 expression in free-electron laser and scalpel incisions during wound healing. *J Invest Dermatol* 2003;**21**:926–32.

CHAPTER 3

The biology of laser–tissue interactions: *in vivo* comparisons and consequences

Peter Whittaker and E Duco Jansen

Introduction

Even after the treatment of more than 10 000 patients with transmyocardial laser revascularization (TMR) over the course of more than 15 years, it is surprising that virtually nothing is known about what tissue effects are required in order to achieve the observed benefit. One prevalent attitude has been, "it works in patients, so there is no need to understand why it works." In fact, it could be argued that the clinical success of TMR has hindered systematic experimental study of potentially crucial laser–tissue effects and hence has delayed, or perhaps even prevented, the discovery of the mechanism(s) of action, thereby potentially hindering improvement or optimization of the procedure.

There is no doubt that during the channel making process lasers produce many different tissue effects that can be altered by changing laser-related parameters. For example, changing the wavelength and the amount of energy delivered has profound consequences on outcome. Some of the effects produced, such as the thermally mediated coagulation and necrosis of muscle cells, appear, on first consideration, to be so obviously "bad" that the laser irradiation parameters should be adjusted so that these effects are eliminated or minimized. More detailed consideration suggests, however, that the circumstances are complex and there may be reasons why such "bad" effects are, in fact, potentially good (or at least not so bad). Nevertheless, these issues have not been examined or, apart from some partisan support for one company's laser system versus another, rarely even considered. Therefore, the aim of this chapter is to examine some of the potential advantages and disadvantages of several laser–tissue interactions, how they might be altered, and which approach would offer the best way of accomplishing the desired result. The major problem we face in such discussion is that the optimal tissue result is unknown and hence we can only offer speculation rather than firm conclusions.

The main difficulty encountered when addressing the optimization of laser parameters is that laser–tissue interactions have received little attention in TMR. When they have been considered, it has been primarily from an engineering and physics perspective [1–3] rather than from a clinical viewpoint. In addition, communication between surgeons, laser manufacturers, and the scientists conducting basic research and preclinical testing has not always occurred. The net result has been that although there is some general awareness that manipulation of laser operating parameters can change the effects on the tissue, there has been no systematic attempt to evaluate the result of altering such parameters and hence no attempt to optimize the operating parameters for any specific laser system. We consider four tissue effects: ablation, coagulation, mechanical disruption, and stimulation. Although it is impossible to address each effect in isolation, because of overlap, we will divide the chapter accordingly into separate sections. However, before we can begin to evaluate such tissue effects, we must start with a critique of the histologic approaches used to examine laser–tissue interactions in TMR.

TMR histology

The assessment and interpretation of TMR results is highly dependent upon the methods used and so when examining the tissue changes produced by TMR, it is imperative to use the appropriate histologic methods. As we will illustrate, the use of inappropriate methods can lead not only to failure to detect potentially important changes, but also to the derivation of false conclusions. There are at least three facets of laser–tissue interaction that merit consideration in a discussion of TMR histology: tissue injury, angio/vasculogenesis, and the healing response to laser injury.

Tissue injury

Mirhoseini [4] first proposed using a laser for TMR, rather than the needles originally used, because he believed that by removing tissue without causing extensive collateral damage, the channels would remain open. This hypothesis assumes that needles cause more mechanical damage to the surrounding myocardium than the combination of thermal and mechanical damage produced by lasers. The key factor in supporting or refuting the hypothesis is the ability to detect injury. The most severe mechanical injury, tearing and disruption of the myocardium, is easy to see in histologic sections. Nevertheless, more subtle, but perhaps just as important, mechanically mediated injury is much harder to detect, especially when examining injury produced in *in vitro* studies. For example, damage to the cell membrane (either mechanical or thermal) can compromise the cell's ability to maintain calcium homeostasis and result in cell necrosis by calcium overload. This type of injury will not be apparent in *ex vivo* studies because of the absence of circulating calcium. In contrast, *in vivo*, such damage is revealed as contraction band necrosis (i.e., calcium overload causes hypercontraction within the cell) and can readily be seen in hematoxylin and eosin-stained (H&E) sections. Typically, such injury is found just beyond the obvious thermal or mechanical injury and thus often provides a useful marker for the edge of the injury. Although contraction band necrosis is readily visible with most stains in bright-field illumination, when polarized light is used the

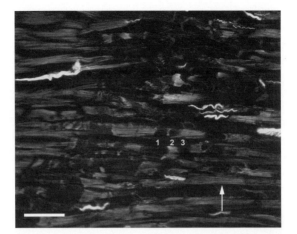

Figure 3.1 Contraction band necrosis adjacent to a laser-made channel (not in the field of view) in a tissue section stained with picrosirius red and viewed with circularly polarized light. The typical appearance of contraction band necrosis is illustrated beneath the numbers. Calcium overload causes hyper-contraction of the cell's contractile elements resulting in a loss of the normal cross-striations (marked by arrow) and their replacement by much wider alternating pattern of dark (1 and 3) and bright (2) regions. Contraction bands of varying widths are present throughout the image. The very bright (and often wavy) structures are collagen fibers. Bar = 35 μm.

contrast between contraction bands and normal tissue is even more striking (Fig. 3.1). In fact, polarized light microscopy has been demonstrated to be effective not only in identifying thermal injury, but also in quantifying the degree of thermal injury [5,6]. Thermal denaturation of muscle and collagen reduces these materials' birefringence and hence thermally injured regions appear darker than normal tissue (Fig. 3.2). We have used this change in the optical properties of thermally injured tissue to determine laser parameters that would minimize thermal injury in a study designed to examine the long-term effect on channel patency and myocardial fibrosis [7]. Similarly, Shehada *et al.* [8] used polarized light microscopy to assess tissue injury after 308 nm xenon chloride excimer laser TMR and evaluate the influence of different operating parameters. Nevertheless, many studies have employed more subjective methods of histologic examination to quantify the extent of thermal injury. Kadipasaoglu *et al.* [9] used a variety of changes including coagulation, contraction bands, and the presence of wavy fibers to assess injury in H&E stained sections and concluded that TMR with a carbon dioxide laser caused 25% less injury than with a xenon chloride excimer laser and 568% less injury than with a holmium:yttrium-aluminium-garnet (YAG) laser.

Obviously, histologic assessment of muscle injury *in vivo* is not possible. Although recent developments in high-resolution optical imaging methods such as optical coherence tomography (OCT) are promising, they have yet to be applied in the field of TMR. Therefore, some groups have measured the release of cardiac enzymes from injured cells in patients as a surrogate marker of cell

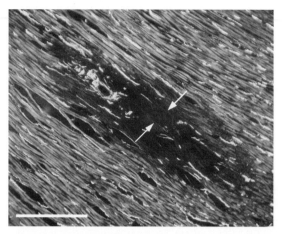

Figure 3.2 Cross-section of a laser channel 1 day after it was made in a rat heart (section stained with picrosirius red and viewed with circularly polarized light). The channel lumen, occluded by thrombus, is located between the arrows. A region of reduced muscle birefringence (i.e., the muscle appears darker than normal), indicative of thermal injury, surrounds the channel. The thermal injury extends further in the direction parallel to the long axis of the cells (top left to bottom right) than in the direction perpendicular to the cells' long axis and hence the region of thermal injury has an ellipsoid shape. Bar = 400 μm.

damage (enzymes have also been measured in animal studies [10]). The results of such studies should, however, be interpreted with caution because it is known that creatine kinase activity is decreased at temperatures greater than 65°C [11]. In addition, muscle coagulation and disruption of blood vessels combined with thermally induced tissue swelling can trap the enzymes within the injured regions limiting their release and hence lead to underestimation of injury.

In summary, there are well-established, quantitative methods available for the histologic assessment of thermal injury that will permit accurate comparison of different TMR methods; however, these have not always been used. Moreover, while histology is a useful marker of tissue injury, the correlation between histologic markers for TMR and its clinical outcome are far from clear.

Angio/vasculogenesis

The detection and measurement of capillaries in the heart is a topic that has generated a considerable amount of research and also the development of specialized techniques. Nevertheless, few TMR studies have adopted these established methodologies. Mueller *et al.* [12] measured vascular density (of both capillaries and arterioles) in porcine hearts 28 days after TMR using a holmium:YAG laser versus that found at the same time after myocardial infarction produced by coronary artery occlusion. In sections cut perpendicular to the channel axis, vascular density was measured in three regions: the channel-associated scar, and two zones of tissue surrounding the channels, one 0.5 mm wide and the other 2 mm wide. Interestingly, vascular density was significantly greater within the laser scar than in the coronary occlusion-induced scar. In contrast, there was no increase in the number of vessels in the non-infarcted myocardium surrounding the channels. The capillary density determined in the normal myocardium, approximately 5 per square millimeter, falls somewhat below the 2–3000 capillaries per square millimeter generally accepted to be the actual myocardial value [13]. Although it might be argued that relative differences measured in such studies are valid, the magnitude of the density shortfall in normal tissue indicates that the method is inadequate and the results obtained may be of limited value. Unfortunately, many other TMR studies have similarly failed to obtain appropriate capillary density values in the control tissue and/or report vascular density per "high-power field" (rather than per square millimeter) or in "arbitrary units," which prevents comparison between studies. Hughes *et al.* [14] examined angiogenesis after TMR with holmium:YAG, carbon dioxide, and xenon-chloride (XeCl) excimer lasers in a pig model of coronary artery stenosis. Although the comparative study design had the potential to reveal interesting information, the method of capillary detection (alkaline phosphatase staining of frozen sections with the muscle cut longitudinally) was flawed and the results were presented in "arbitrary units." With such staining, the muscle should be cut in cross-section to reveal capillary density [15]. The majority of capillaries run parallel to the muscle cells' long axis and so to examine tissue in which the cells are cut longitudinally provides few useful data. Furthermore, using such longitudinally sectioned tissue, the apparent capillary density can be significantly influenced by slight variations in sectioning plane; it is clear from the examples shown in this particular study that the sectioning plane did indeed differ between samples. The authors concluded that holimium:YAG and carbon dioxide lasers produced an increase in capillary density versus both XeCl excimer laser treatment and control [14]; however, for the reasons stated, that conclusion appears suspect.

Moreover, it is also difficult to see how capillary density can be increased above the normal values; at approximately 2–3000 per square millimeter – there is little extra space available. In addition, theoretical models, based on oxygen diffusion distances, indicate that such densities represent the optimum configuration. We compared capillary density, using standard methods [16], 2 months after TMR with either a 26-gauge hypodermic syringe needle or a holmium:YAG laser coupled to a 400-µm diameter optic fiber in normal rat hearts and found no increase after TMR with either device versus untreated control myocardium [7]. On the other hand, in cases of muscle cell hypertrophy (a probable feature in TMR-treated patients), oxygen diffusion distances would be increased and additional capillaries would have value; however, most TMR studies have not used animal models in which hypertrophy is present.

It could also be argued that an increase in capillary density is of little value if the number of larger vessels that feed blood flow into the capillaries is not increased. For example, if capillary density increased but vascular density, and hence blood supply, remained the same, then the only effect would be a redistribution of the same flow. Although redistribution may have some benefit (e.g., a shift from subepicardial to subendocardial flow could, under certain circumstances, be useful), the original goal of TMR was to increase flow. Hence, evaluation of changes in the density of larger vessels may be a more appropriate parameter to consider. Although Mueller *et al.* [12,17] reported no increase in arteriolar density in tissue adjacent to TMR channels versus untreated tissue, other investigators have found increased numbers of smooth muscle-containing blood vessels in tissue adjacent to TMR scars (e.g., with a holmium:YAG laser) [18]. Nevertheless, unless these larger vessels bring blood flow from a different source (i.e., from the ventricular cavity or another, non-ischemic, part of the heart rather than from the original diseased coronary artery), as was also the case with the Vineberg procedure in which the internal mammary artery was tunneled into the myocardial, then an increase in vascular density will only succeed in redistributing rather than increasing blood flow.

Therefore, based on the published literature, which has used, for the most part, flawed methodology, it is impossible to come to any conclusion regarding which, if any, laser (or set of laser parameters) results in the greatest increase in vascular density. In fact, it is unclear if TMR is associated with any increase in vascular density in tissue surrounding the channels.

Healing

The qualitative examination of scar tissue produced after the channels are made has been a component of many studies. Most of these have been primarily interested in whether or not the scar tissue has infiltrated into the original ablation channel and occluded it. Such studies clearly do not need sophisticated methods of histologic analysis to distinguish open versus closed. Nevertheless, one feature of potential importance to the long-term effect of TMR on cardiac function is whether or not creation of the channels provokes an increase in collagen content away from the channel or channel scar. It is well known that myocardial infarction results, over the subsequent weeks to months, in an increase in interstitial collagen content in the remaining viable myocardium distant from the healed infarct. The presence of additional collagen adversely affects cardiac function by increasing myocardial stiffness, which can hinder both systolic and diastolic function, and by blocking electrical signal propagation, which can lead to the genesis of arrhythmias such as ventricular tachycardia. TMR can be considered to produce many mini-infarcts and so it would be reasonable to expect that similar fibrotic changes might occur. Indeed, we found in our long-term study that collagen content was significantly increased in the left ventricular free-wall after holmium:YAG, but not after needle TMR [7].

The histologic detection and identification of collagen has traditionally been achieved with trichrome staining; however, this method has limitations. The precise staining mechanism is still a subject of debate and it is a notoriously difficult stain to obtain consistent results with. In addition, we have found that although trichrome readily identifies thick collagen fibers, it is poor at staining thin fibers and hence can underestimate collagen content. For example, we found that myocardial collagen content was consistently lower (by as much as

300%) measured in trichrome-stained sections versus that measured from serial sections stained with picrosirius red and viewed with polarized light [19]. Most TMR studies do not use picrosirius red staining and hence it would not be surprising if increases in collagen had been overlooked. For instance, Domkowski *et al.* [20] examined tissue from a patient who died 9 months after TMR with a carbon dioxide laser and reported, on the basis of trichrome staining, minimal scarring in myocardium surrounding the channels.

The detection of collagen is a neglected but potentially important facet of histologic analysis in TMR because of the impact that increased interstitial fibrosis can have on cardiac function and on arrhythmia. The limited available data suggest that TMR, at least with holmium:YAG lasers, can increase myocardial collagen content away from the channels.

Tissue ablation

The mechanisms of laser–tissue interaction at different wavelengths strongly influence the ablation process in TMR and have been discussed in some detail for lasers in general [3] and also for carbon dioxide lasers specifically [2] in previous reviews. Briefly, infrared lasers produce ablation through absorption of energy by water within the tissue, while ultraviolet energy is absorbed directly by chemical bonds within protein molecules. Thus, there is no doubt that ablation of myocardium can be achieved by many kinds of lasers. In fact, even laser wavelengths that have not been used clinically for TMR such as 1064 and 532 nm can, if the pulse width is sufficiently short, produce ablation. Such manipulation of pulse width to alter the laser–tissue interaction is an important point because continuous wave neodymium:YAG lasers (wavelength 1064 nm) have often been used to coagulate, rather than vaporize, myocardial tissue for the treatment of ventricular arrhythmias [21]. In contrast, Ogura *et al.* [22] also used a neodymium:YAG laser, but with a pulse frequency of 10 Hz and with each pulse less than 10 ns in duration, to produce myocardial channels; ablation was more efficient and the adjacent thermal injury (detected using polarized light microscopy) less with the 1064 nm wavelength than at 532 nm. It is noteworthy that the underlying mechanisms leading to ablation with these parameters are fundamentally different in that they are dependent on the formation of a laser-induced plasma and subsequent ionization of the material. Although comparison of the results obtained with those from other studies is compromised because this *in vitro* experiment was conducted on cooled tissue (3°C), this study illustrates that TMR with lasers other than those currently used in clinical practice is possible.

A further caveat should be added because the majority of ablation studies have examined the effect in normal animal hearts. This is potentially important because the energy required to ablate muscle and collagen is different. Theoretically, on this basis, a case could be made for ultraviolet lasers being more effective for ablating the fibrotic myocardial tissue likely to be present in patients requiring TMR. Nevertheless, if open channels are not required in order to achieve clinical benefit, then tissue ablation may be unnecessary.

Coagulation

Myocardial coagulation produced by tissue heating offers several potential explanations for TMR-related benefits. For example, coagulation may be beneficial because it reduces the number of muscle cells within the underperfused region and hence favorably alters the supply : demand ratio even if blood flow is not increased. In addition, extensive coagulation is likely to increase the amount of nerve damage and hence perhaps reduce the amount of perceived anginal pain. Furthermore, a larger necrotic region may stimulate the growth of additional blood vessels to implement healing. Although the growth of such new vessels to supply the developing scar may not directly benefit the surrounding muscle, it is possible that favorable blood flow redistribution may, as discussed earlier, occur as a result of such vasculogenesis.

The extent of thermal coagulation surrounding the channels is influenced not only by wavelength, but also by other laser parameters including pulse energy, pulse length, pulse repetition rate, and beam size/profile. The influence of such parameters has, however, not been examined in a systematic manner and so it is difficult to make definitive conclusions about which lasers produce more or less coagulation. It is generally true to say that ultraviolet lasers produce less thermal coagulation than infrared lasers; however, it is also certainly possible to alter the irradiation parameters such that an ultraviolet laser produces a large amount of coagulation or, conversely, that an infrared laser produces a small amount of coagulation. For example, we found a high channel patency (89%) with a small amount of surrounding scar tissue ($145 \pm 10 \, \mu m$) in rat hearts several months after TMR with a frequency-tripled neodymium:YAG laser (wavelength 355 nm) and a pulse energy of 10 mJ; however, when the pulse energy was reduced to 5 mJ, the patency was reduced (46%) and the amount of scar tissue was increased by 50% ($220 \pm 25 \, \mu m$) [23]. Shehada et al. [8] found that the amount of thermal injury produced in pig hearts using a 308-nm excimer laser varied considerably with pulse repetition rate, fiber diameter, and the advancement rate of the fiber through the tissue even when the radiant exposure was kept constant. They concluded that the variation of these parameters allowed a significant amount of flexibility in the creation of channel morphology and surrounding coagulation. The fact that such flexibility was achieved using a single wavelength indicates that it would be unwise to make the generalization that one type of laser is better or worse than another. In fact, it is probable that the operating parameters of any laser could be altered in such a way to produce a lesion of any desired configuration.

Another issue that is of potential importance for coagulation is that the data obtained from the published animal studies may well overestimate the amount of injury in patients. This is because the animal studies have, for the most part, been conducted on normal, healthy adult (or even juvenile) subjects versus the diseased and typically older clinical subjects. Hearts from the latter group will be more fibrotic than those from the former cohort. The presence of fibrosis can limit the extent of thermal injury surrounding TMR channels. In Figure 3.3,

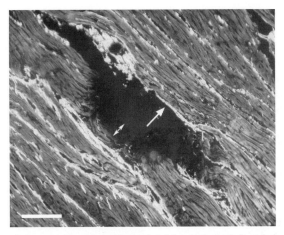

Figure 3.3 Channel cross-section (picrosirius red staining and circularly polarized light) showing asymmetrical thermal injury in the presence of collagen fibers. There is no thermal injury (reduction in brightness) to the muscle above the thick bundle of collagen fibers on one side of the channel (marked by arrow). In contrast, on the opposite side of the channel, there is a band of thermally injured muscle approximately 100 μm wide (marked by the double headed arrow). The presence of collagen provided a barrier to the propagation of thermal injury. Bar = 250 μm.

collagen fibers adjacent to the channel protected muscle cells immediately above from coagulation. In contrast, there was thermal injury to the muscle on the opposite side of the channel. In the same way that collagen fibers can block the electrical conduction, they can also provide a barrier to heat propagation. Thus, in hearts with greater amounts of interstitial fibrosis, there may be less thermal injury to the muscle. This suggestion is supported by evidence from examination of human tissue. For example, a study using an argon laser to coagulate samples of human myocardium found that in order to produce thermal lesions in the diseased tissue of a similar size as those in normal hearts, a higher energy was required [24].

In addition to muscle necrosis, thermal coagulation has the potential to kill nerve fibers. For instance, a small clinical study examined the effect of both holmium:YAG and excimer laser TMR on cardiac innervation using iodine-123-labeled meta-iodobenzylguanide (MIBG), which is taken up by sympathetic nerve endings and hence allows scintigraphic identification of the cardiac sympathetic nervous system [25]. Overall, there was a decrease in MIBG uptake in the laser-treated regions when assessed 1 month after TMR and denervation was still observed 16 months later. Nevertheless, denervation was found in only 45% of the treated segments even though all of the patients experienced a reduction of 2 or more in their New York Heart Association class. The small sample size makes definitive conclusions impossible; however, there was no apparent difference in the results obtained for the two laser systems used and so we are unable to determine whether there is more merit in one approach than the other. The subepicardial location of the bulk of the sympathetic nerve fibers [26] suggests that the transmural coagulation achieved with TMR has a much greater opportunity to damage or kill nerve fibers than the subendocardial coagulation that will occur after percutaneous myocardial revascularization (PMR). Indeed, one PMR study concluded that the procedure was successful (the patients' Canadian Cardiovascular Society score decreased from 3.0 ± 0.8 to 1.9 ± 0.9 at 1 month; $P < 0.01$) in the absence of any detectable sign of denervation [27]. The latter study also implies that denervation may not be necessary to achieve clinical success.

Although the issue of the eventual reduction in volume of the coagulated muscle as the scar shrinks is one that has received little attention, it is one that has potential significance. The major structural changes that occur were quantified by Fisher *et al.* [28] in a study comparing the effects of carbon dioxide and holmium:YAG lasers. These investigators found, using serial sectioning of tissue obtained at 6 hours to 6 weeks after TMR in normal dog hearts, that although the volume of acute (6 hours) injury was three times greater after holmium:YAG than after carbon dioxide laser TMR, there was little volume difference between groups at 6 weeks. Furthermore, the eventual scar volume reduction was 86% with carbon dioxide and 93% with holmium:YAG. This study demonstrates not only the considerable reduction in volume, but also that large volumes of thermal injury shrink proportionately more than smaller volumes.

This local cardiac remodeling has potential architectural consequences that extend beyond the scar. First, there is the obvious possible contribution to channel closure. If the initial thrombotic channel occlusion is resolved, then the subsequent shrinkage in the tissue surrounding the channel appears likely to, at best, reduce channel width and, at worst, completely eliminate the channel. On the other hand, there is also a possible beneficial effect. The combined shrinkage contribution of 30–40 transmural channels may be sufficient to decrease ventricular volume in hearts that were initially dilated; essentially performing a Batista procedure without excision. We are unaware of any study that has examined this possibility either in animals or humans. Conversely, scar shrinkage could result in adverse myocardial remodeling; for example, muscle cell disarray similar to that seen in cases of hypertrophic cardiomyopathy has been found adjacent to holmium:YAG-produced fibrosis [7]. Another possible outcome of tissue shrinkage is the likelihood that it could confound interpretation of blood flow measurement within the treated region. The majority of studies that have examined blood flow in patients have used nuclear methods, which involve dividing ventricular cross-sections into segments. The before and after TMR comparisons that are made assume that the before and after images can be superimposed. If shrinkage has occurred, then such assumptions may not be valid and normally perfused tissue (or at least tissue that had not been considered worthy of treatment) that had previously been outside of the "hypoperfused" region may now have been pulled inside and hence give the impression that blood flow has been increased.

The amount of coagulation produced by the different laser systems most often used in TMR indicates that there is more tissue shrinkage with the holmium:YAG than with the carbon dioxide laser. Although the ultraviolet XeCl excimer laser theoretically has the capability of causing little coagulation (even though the total amount of damage may be significant, largely because of explosive mechanical effects similar to those seen during laser angioplasty), the system used by one of the manufacturers, Acculase, Inc., caused the optical fiber to rotate so that a channel larger than the diameter of the fiber was created. This approach also increased coagulation to the surrounding tissue; for example, micrographs in the paper by Mack *et al.* [29] of channels made in sheep hearts show significant thermal injury. In addition, one clinical study using this device [30] created more channels than is typical; 69 ± 5 channels attempted per patient versus the 30–40 usually made in studies using carbon dioxide lasers. Such a large number of channels increases the potential for appreciable tissue shrinkage. Therefore, again there is no conclusive evidence to support the selection of one laser over another.

Furthermore, if coagulation, no matter the extent, is the parameter solely responsible for the clinical benefit, then there is no need for a laser. Coagulation is easily achieved using simpler and less expensive devices; for example, radio-frequency probes and even hot needles have been used in animal studies. Interestingly, the former approach has also been shown to be associated with both myocardial angiogenesis and denervation [31]. The authors of the study concluded that radio-frequency energy might provide a viable alternative to laser TMR.

Potential confounding factors

As if comparison between TMR studies were not difficult enough, there are some additional experimental factors that have the potential to confound further interpretation of the data. Specifically, there are factors that could protect muscle cells from thermal injury and hence limit the amount of damage. For example, *in vitro*, it is possible that sample temperature at the time of testing could limit the extent of thermal injury. Such *in vitro* testing is frequently performed on tissue obtained from abattoirs, which is often stored in cold saline until the experiments are carried out. If the tissue is not then warmed to body temperature, the extent of coagulation will be reduced. A corollary to this effect may also occur in clinical practice when TMR is combined with bypass graft surgery. For example, Loubani *et al.* [32] combined bypass and intermittent cross-clamp fibrillation with mild hypothermia (32°C) and then made channels in non-graftable regions of the heart with a holmium:YAG laser. It seems likely that the extent of thermal injury would be less under these circumstances than in the absence of hypothermia; however, this possibility has not been examined.

It is also possible that the choice of anesthetic may influence cell injury because some agents are known to exert cardioprotective effects. For example, fentanyl has been shown to produce a significant decrease in infarct size associated with both a 90-minute coronary artery occlusion in dogs [33] and after 20 minutes of global ischemia in rat hearts [34] and was attributed to activation of δ-opioid receptors and protein kinase C. Furthermore, halogenated anesthetics, such as isoflurane and halothane, in addition to morphine and propofol, also exert protection against ischemic injury (reviewed in Kato and Foëx [35]). Although these agents are sometimes used in experimental studies, they are much more commonly used clinically; however, whether or not these agents can also protect against thermally mediated cell injury has yet to be examined.

An additional potential source of cardioprotection that may influence the extent of muscle injury is ischemic preconditioning; that is, the phenomenon whereby brief periods of transient ischemia prior to a longer, sustained ischemic period reduce the amount of cell death [36]. To ensure that channels are made in the appropriate location (i.e., in the tissue that will subsequently be made ischemic), several studies have used brief coronary artery occlusions to identify, either by tissue blanching or dyskenesis, this target region [9,37]. However, this approach may be sufficient to precondition the tissue and hence reduce the amount of cell injury. Although the mechanism of the preconditioning-mediated protection is not yet fully understood, there is compelling evidence that signal transduction pathways involving G-coupled proteins, protein kinase C, and tyrosine kinases all have a role [36]. It is interesting to note that some of these same pathways are also involved in the stimulation of angiogenesis [38]. Thus, the use of brief coronary artery occlusion to delineate the tissue bed where the channels will be made can not only exert protection, but may also help provoke angiogenesis. Ischemic preconditioning has been deliberately used as a protective mechanism in at least one study combining bypass graft surgery with TMR [39]. Five-minute occlusions of the left anterior descending artery or right coronary artery followed by 5 minutes of reperfusion were made prior to the bypass procedure. Although TMR was performed before ischemic preconditioning in most of the treated patients (and hence the intent was to protect the heart during vascular anastomosis rather than to protect against TMR-mediated injury), in cases where distal segments of the bypassed artery were completely occluded, the graft was anastomosed to the proximal segment and TMR performed afterwards in the distal tissue bed. Unfortunately, the patients treated in this manner were not analyzed separately and so we cannot determine if preconditioning provided protection.

The influences of tissue temperature, anesthetic, and ischemic preconditioning not only have the potential to limit the amount of thermal injury, but also provide three additional variables that must be considered when TMR study comparisons are made. Nevertheless, despite the well-known cardioprotective effects of these factors, they have yet to be evaluated in any TMR experiments.

Mechanical disruption of tissue

This phenomenon, produced because gas bubbles formed during ablation may be unable to escape up the portion of the channel already created, appears likely to be detrimental. A similar effect has been described in laser angioplasty with both pulsed XeCl excimer and pulsed infrared lasers [40,41]. The tissue can be badly torn as the bubbles track along the path of least resistance; that is, parallel to the long axis of the muscle cells. This effect creates flaps of myocardial tissue, typically at the lateral edges of elliptical channels [42]. It is likely that such mechanical injury will also result in necrosis of that muscle, even if it was not coagulated by thermal injury, and can extend a significant distance from the channel. Moreover, the expanding vapor cavity may facilitate rapid convective transfer of heat to regions well beyond those that may be expected to be heated based on optical parameters or heat diffusion [2]. Healing of this type of injury will result in increased amounts of interstitial collagen between viable muscle cells, which often appears as long arms of fibrosis extending perpendicularly from the original channel (Fig. 3.4). As discussed, not only will this additional fibrosis adversely affect systolic and diastolic function by making the hearts stiffer, but also will affect the transverse propagation of electrical signals.

A good case could be made for this being the TMR laser–tissue interaction most useful to avoid. It is unlikely that there is much to gain from this structural change; however, there appears to be much to lose. The use of holmium:YAG lasers appears to be associated with the greatest extent of such injury, although significant mechanical injury has also been seen with excimer lasers. In contrast, the high-power carbon dioxide laser produces less damage, presumably because the pulse duration associated with this latter approach is typically 2–3 orders of magnitude longer hence resulting in a less explosive event [2]. The disruption of normal myocardial architecture with its subsequent potential for adverse effects on cardiac function and electrical conduction, while not immediately catastrophic, represents a long-term danger. We are unaware of any reports documenting such complications; however, the length of time required for them to become apparent is unknown and the long-term follow-up studies that have been conducted have not examined histology.

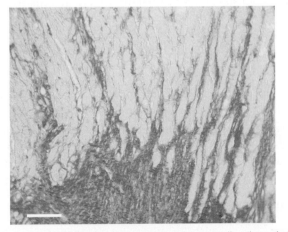

Figure 3.4 Channel-associated fibrosis extending into the surrounding tissue (rat heart stained with picrosirius red and view with bright-field illumination). The original laser channel was made from left to right at the bottom of the image. Bands of fibrosis (the darker material) extend perpendicular to the channel's long axis for several hundred μm separating previously adjacent myocytes. Bar = 100 μm.

As with thermal coagulation, mechanical disruption or mechanically in-duced tissue necrosis are not events that are exclusive to lasers. Several studies have demonstrated that the angiogenic response to devices that induce me-chanical injury is similar to that produced by lasers. For example, Chu *et al.* [43] found a significant increase in both neovascularization and in immunohisto-chemically detected vascular endothelial growth factor and basic fibroblast growth factor in pig hearts after transmural channels were made using an 18-gauge hypodermic needle. Similarly, Malekan *et al.* [44] found no difference in channel scar appearance 4 weeks after their creation in sheep hearts with either a carbon dioxide laser or a mechanical power drill.

Stimulation

In this context, we do not mean the potential stimulating effects of thermal or mechanical injury surrounding the channels, but rather the direct stimulating effect of laser irradiation. Scattering of photons by tissue elements results in the incident beam extending beyond the zone of thermal injury; however, in such regions the energy will be so low that there will be negligible heating. This situ-ation is analogous to so-called low-level laser therapy, in which low-power (typ-ically <100 mW) red or infrared lasers are used to treat a wide variety of diseases. Although this field is controversial because of the claims that it is a panacea, there is nevertheless evidence that low-power laser irradiation can indeed exert cellular effects, most probably because of cytochrome-mediated absorption of light in cellular organelles such as mitochondria [45]. The significant absorption of ultraviolet radiation by hemoglobin limits the possibility that either the ex-cimer or frequency-tripled neodymium:YAG lasers would exert such an effect. The significant water absorption of 10 600 nm radiation similarly means that the carbon dioxide laser is also unlikely to exert a stimulating effect via this mecha-nism. There is also strong absorption by water at the wavelength of the holmi-um:YAG (2100 nm) and the neodymium:YAG (1064 nm) lasers; however, some transmission is likely beyond the zone of thermal injury. Low-level laser thera-py has been suggested to accelerate wound healing, produce angiogenesis, and alleviate pain, which could all have a role in explaining treatment effects report-ed after TMR. Nevertheless, it is difficult, if not impossible, to attribute such changes solely to low-level laser irradiation because these parameters are also affected by other facets of TMR as discussed earlier. Furthermore, such benefits are usually associated with long-term biologic effects and thus it is difficult to see how the reported immediate benefits can be explained by these mechanisms.

Conclusions

As stated at the beginning of the chapter, our lack of understanding of the mech-anism of TMR makes it impossible to be definitive in any conclusion. Nevert he-less, after consideration of the above discussion of laser–tissue interactions, it is

difficult to imagine why a laser would be necessary for TMR. Mirhosieni's original rational for using the carbon dioxide laser was that it would cause less damage to the tissue surrounding the channel than the mechanical methods that had
been used earlier. That hypothesis is clearly not supported by the data when
appropriate methods are used to reveal the actual extent of thermal injury surrounding the channels. Furthermore, we have seen that although lasers can cut,
coagulate, and mechanically disrupt the myocardium these properties are
not exclusive to lasers. Indeed, numerous other devices ranging from radio-
frequency probes to hypodermic needles and even power drills were able to
achieve similar results to those obtained with lasers in animal TMR studies and
have a potentially significant advantage over lasers in that they are usually
simpler and cheaper. Even the more nebulous possible mechanism of light-
mediated cellular stimulation could likely be achieved using light-emitting
diodes rather than lasers. Furthermore, comparison of the results obtained in
different TMR studies is confounded not only by the large number of variables
related to laser operation (e.g., pulse width, pulse repetition rate, beam profile)
that have been used, but also by the different experimental conditions (animal
models, tissue temperature, anesthesia, ischemic preconditioning) that have
been employed and sometimes not adequately reported. It is therefore not surprising that we appear to be no closer to understanding the mechanism of action
of TMR than we were 15 years ago.

References

1 McKenzie AL. Physics of thermal processes in laser–tissue interaction. *Phys Med Biol*
1990;**35**:1175–209.
2 Jansen ED, Frenz M, Kadipasaoglu KA, *et al*. Laser–tissue interaction during transmyocardial laser revascularization. *Ann Thorac Surg* 1997;**63**:640–7.
3 Hartman RA, Whittaker P. The physics of transmyocardial laser revascularization. *J Clin
Laser Med Surg* 1997;**15**:255–9.
4 Mirhoseini M, Cayton MM. Three decades of experience: transmyocardial laser revascularization. In: Okada M (ed.) *Current Topics in Transmyocardial Laser Revascularization*. Tokyo,
Japan: Medical Tribune, 2001: 203–32.
5 Thomsen S, Pierce JA, Cheong WF. Changes in birefringence as markers of thermal injury in
tissues. *IEEE Trans Biomed Eng* 1989;**36**:1174–9.
6 Whittaker P, Zheng S, Patterson MJ, *et al*. Histologic signatures of thermal injury: applications in transmyocardial laser revascularization and radiofrequency ablation. *Lasers Surg
Med* 2000;**27**:305–18.
7 Whittaker P, Rakusan K, Kloner RA. Transmural channels can protect ischemic tissue: assessment of long-term myocardial response to laser- and needle-made channels. *Circulation*
1996;**93**:143–52.
8 Shehada REN, Papaioannou T, Mansour HN, Grundfest WS. Excimer laser (308 nm) based
transmyocardium laser revascularization: effects of the lasing parameters on myocardial
histology. *Lasers Surg Med* 2001;**29**:85–91.
9 Kadipasaoglu KA, Pehlivanoglu S, Conger JL, *et al*. Long- and short-term effects of
transmyocardial laser revascularization in acute myocardial ischemia. *Lasers Surg Med*
1997;**20**:6–14.

10 Kitade T, Okada M, Tsuji Y, Nakamura M, Matoba Y. Experimental investigations on relationships between myocardial damage and laser type used in transmyocardial laser revascularization (TMLR). *Kobe J Med Sci* 1999;**45**:127–36.

11 Haines DE, Whayne JG, Walker J, Nath S, Bruns DE. The effect of radiofrequency catheter ablation on myocardial creatine kinase activity. *J Cardiovasc Electrophysiol* 1995;**6**:79–88.

12 Mueller XM, Tevaearai HT, Genton C-Y, Chaubert P, von Segesser LK. Improved neoangiogenesis in transmyocardial laser revascularization combined with angiogenic adjunct in a pig model. *Clin Sci* 2000;**99**:535–40.

13 Rakusan K, Heron MI, Kolar F, Korecky B. Transplantation-induced atrophy of normal and hypertrophic rat hearts: effect on cardiac myocytes and capillaries. *J Mol Cell Cardiol* 1997;**29**:1045–54.

14 Hughes GC, Kypson AP, Annex BH, *et al.* Induction of angiogenesis after TMR: a comparison of holmium:YAG, CO_2, and excimer lasers. *Ann Thorac Surg* 2000;**70**:504–9.

15 Przyklenk K, Groom AC. Can exercise promote revascularization in the transition zone of infracted rat hearts? *Can J Physiol Pharmacol* 1984;**62**:630–3.

16 Rakusan K, Turek Z. Protamine inhibits capillary formation in growing rat hearts. *Circ Res* 1985;**57**:393–8.

17 Mueller XM, Tevaearai HT, Genton C-Y, Chaubert P, von Segesser LK. Are there vascular density gradients along myocardial laser channels? *Ann Thorac Surg* 1999;**68**:125–30.

18 Yamamoto N, Kohmoto T, Gu A, *et al.* Angiogenesis is enhanced in ischemic canine myocardium by transmyocardial laser revascularization. *J Am Coll Cardiol* 1998;**31**: 1426–33.

19 Whittaker P, Kloner RA, Boughner DR, Pickering JG. Quantitative assessment of myocardial collagen with picrosirius red staining and circularly polarized light. *Basic Res Cardiol* 1994;**89**:397–410.

20 Domkowski PW, Biswas SS, Steenbergen C, Lowe JE. Histological evidence of angiogenesis 9 months after transmyocardial laser revascularization. *Circulation* 2001;**103**:469–71.

21 Weber HP, Heinze A, Enders S, Ruprecht L, Unsöld E. Laser catheter coagulation of normal and scarred ventricular myocardium in dogs. *Lasers Surg Med* 1998;**22**:109–19.

22 Ogura M, Sato S, Ishihara M, *et al.* Myocardium tissue ablation with high-peak-power nanosecond 1,064- and 532-nm pulsed lasers: influence of laser-induced plasma. *Lasers Surg Med* 2002;**31**:136–41.

23 Whittaker P, Spariosu K, Ho ZZ. Success of transmyocardial laser revascularization is determined by the amount and organization of scar tissue produced in response to initial injury: results of ultraviolet laser treatment. *Lasers Surg Med* 1999;**24**:253–60.

24 Saksena S, Ciccone JM, Chandran P, *et al.* Laser ablation of normal and diseased human ventricle. *Am Heart J* 1986;**112**:52–60.

25 Beek JF, van der Sloot JAP, Huikeshoven M, *et al.* Cardiac denervation after clinical transmyocardial laser revascularization: short-term and long-term iodine 123-labeled metaiodobenzylguanide scintigraphic evidence. *J Thorac Cardiovasc Surg* 2004;**127**:517–24.

26 Barber MJ, Mueller TM, Davies BG, Zipes DP. Phenol topically applied to canine left ventricular epicardium interrupts sympathetic but not vagal afferents. *Circ Res* 1984;**55**:532–44.

27 Guzzetti S, Colombo A, Piccaluga E, *et al.* Absence of clinical signs of cardiac denervation after percutaneous myocardial laser revascularization. *Int J Cardiol* 2003;**91**:129–35.

28 Fisher PE, Khomoto T, DeRosa CM, *et al.* Histologic analysis of transmyocardial channels: comparison of CO_2 and holmium:YAG lasers. *Ann Thorac Surg* 1997;**64**:466–72.

29 Mack CA, Magovern CJ, Hahn RT, *et al.* Channel patency and neovascularization after transmyocardial revascularization using an excimer laser: results and comparisons to non-laser channels. *Circulation* 1997;**96**(Suppl 2):65–9.

30 Kavanagh GJ, Whittaker P, Prejean CA Jr, *et al.* Dissociation between improvement in angina pectoris and myocardial perfusion after transmyocardial revascularization with an excimer laser. *Am J Cardiol* 2001;**87**:229–31.

31 Yamamoto N, Gu A, DeRosa CM, *et al.* Radio frequency transmyocardial revascularization enhances angiogenesis and causes myocardial denervation in canine model. *Lasers Surg Med* 2000;**27**:18–28.

32 Loubani M, Chin D, Leverment JN, Galiñanes M. Mid-term results of combined transmyocardial laser revascularization and coronary artery bypass. *Ann Thorac Surg* 2003;**76**:1163–6.

33 Mergner GW, Mergner WJ, Stoiko M. Anesthetics influence myocardial infarct size. *Adv Myocardiol* 1985;**6**:593–606.

34 Kato R, Foëx P. Fentanyl reduces infarction but not stunning via _-opioid receptors and protein kinase C in rats. *Br J Anaesth* 2000;**84**:608–14.

35 Kato R, Foëx P. Myocardial protection by anesthetic agents against ischemia-reperfusion injury: an update for anesthesiologists. *Can J Anesth* 2002;**49**:777–91.

36 Przyklenk K, Kloner RA. Ischemic preconditioning: exploring the paradox. *Prog Cardiovasc Dis* 1998;**40**:517–47.

37 Yano OJ, Bielefeld MR, Jeevanandam V, *et al.* Prevention of acute regional ischemia with endocardial laser channels. *Ann Thorac Surg* 1993;**56**:46–53.

38 Idris I, Gray S, Donnelly R. Protein kinase C activation: isoenzyme-specific effects on metabolism and cardiovascular complications in diabetes. *Diabetologia* 2001;**44**:659–73.

39 Trehan N, Mishra M, Bapna R, *et al.* Transmyocardial laser revascularization combined with coronary artery bypass grafting without cardiopulmonary bypass. *Eur J Cardiothorac Surg* 1997;**12**:276–84.

40 van Leeuwen TG, Meertens JH, Velema E, Post MJ, Borst C. Intraluminal vapor bubble induced by excimer laser pulse causes microsecond arterial dilation and invagination leading to extensive wall damage in the rabbit. *Circulation* 1993;**87**:1258–63.

41 van Erven L, van Leeuwen TG, Post MJ, *et al.* Mid-infrared pulsed laser ablation of the arterial wall. Mechanical origin of "acoustic" wall damage and its effects on wall healing. *J Thorac Surg* 1992;**104**:1053–9.

42 Whittaker P. Detection and assessment of laser-mediated injury in transmyocardial revascularization. *J Clin Laser Med Surg* 1997;**15**:261–7.

43 Chu V, Kuang J-Q, McGinn A, *et al.* Angiogenic response induced by mechanical transmyocardial revascularization. *J Thorac Cardiovasc Surg* 1999;**118**:849–56.

44 Malekan R, Reynolds C, Narula N, *et al.* Angiogenesis in transmyocardila laser revascularization: a non-specific response to injury. *Circulation* 1998;**98**(Suppl 2):62–5.

45 Karu T. Primary and secondary mechanisms of action of visible to near-IR radiation on cells. *J Photochem Photobiol B* 1999;**49**:1–17.

CHAPTER 4

Histopathologic effects of transmyocardial laser revascularization on myocardium: assessment of channel patency

Kamuran A Kadipasaoglu, Egemen Tuzun, and OH Frazier

Introduction

Seldom does the clinical world witness a controversy as intense as the one that, for more than a decade, has surrounded transmyocardial laser revascularization (TMR). The technique has been called terms as contrasting as "a viable alternative to coronary artery bypass graft (CABG)" and "a reptilian fallacy." Perhaps what fuels the controversy is the pitting against each other of the repeated observations of TMR's clinical effect(s) and the lack of objective evidence for a causal relationship tying such effects to the treatment. Not surprisingly, this discrepancy between practice and theory led to speculations that the symptomatic relief following the treatment may be related to placebo effect or tissue denervation. To further the confusion, several laser modalities were adopted for performing the procedure, each with its idiosyncratic tissue interaction patterns and channel morphology, and its associated financial interest groups.

As is the case with every investigational device, prospective users and governing agencies are interested primarily in the safety and efficacy of TMR. Technically speaking, cardiac perfusion is the most relevant endpoint that would provide unequivocal proof of clinical efficacy. Cardiac perfusion is objective and quantitative, and any other variable is secondary to it, including cardiac function, exercise tolerance, quality of life, and symptomatic changes. Unfortunately, there is no current diagnostic technology that can measure the absolute change in cardiac perfusion with acceptable accuracy and sensitivity. Historically, randomized clinical trials that chose cardiac perfusion as the primary endpoint have been criticized on the grounds that sample size was too small, study design precluded prospective randomization, diagnostic technique was inaccurate/insensitive, confounding effect(s) such as adjunctive CABG were present, or, simply, that the outcome was negative. Safety, on the other hand, cannot be as easily tied to a single dependent variable. Freedom from major adverse cardiac events (MACE) is a universally accepted, compounded endpoint for safety, but there are also conflicting results and contradictory reports associated with MACE, which are discussed elsewhere in this book. Therefore, MACE and cardiac perfusion, pivotal parameters for extracting information on safety and efficacy, have been ineffective in building a consensus for TMR. Channel histo-morphology, a secondary endpoint, is equally relevant to the controversy but not as directly critical as cardiac perfusion in establishing a causal relationship between TMR and its effect(s).

Two mechanisms have been proposed through which arterial blood can be carried to the myocardium. According to the first, the newly formed laser chan-nels remain connected to the left ventricular (LV) cavity at the subendocardial level and establish patent links to the native intramyocardial vasculature. These channels would remain patent in the chronic phase and continuously transport intraventricular blood to the submyocardial and mid-myocardial levels. The al-ternative mechanism proposes that the channels themselves occlude but that the healing process causes a significantly large number of vessels to proliferate. If this neovascular network remains connected to the endocardial surface, a fresh supply of blood would be redistributed to the myocardium. If, on the other hand, the neovasculature connects to the epicardial coronary arteries, resistance to anterograde perfusion would be reduced, resulting in increased flow in the coronary vasculature. Of course, any combination of these possibilities is equally imaginable and potentially possible.

Unfortunately, as with the case of cardiac perfusion, the issues remain unre-solved – especially whether transmural channels remain patent and whether they connect to the endocardium or to the native vasculature. There are many differing viewpoints, and it is the purpose of this chapter to elucidate some of the arguments. We begin with an introductory discussion of the human my-ocardial vasculature and laser–tissue interactions.

Blood supply of human and reptilian hearts

The coronary arterial system is the principal route for delivery of oxygenated blood to the myocardium. However, following occlusion of one of the coronary arteries, blood may be supplied to the ischemic myocardium by accessory path-ways, the so-called "coronary collateral circulation" (Fig. 4.1). The collateral cir-culation may be subdivided into two major anatomic groups: intracardiac and extracardiac anastomoses. The intracardiac anastomoses consist of interatrial and endomural channels, while the extracardiac anastomoses consist of retro-cardiac and transepicardial communications [1].

Direct communication between the coronary arteries and heart's chambers (arterioluminal channels) was first described by Vieussens [2] in 1706. Two years later, Thebesius [3] identified direct connections between coronary veins and the cavities of the heart. In 1933, arteriosinusoidal channels, another type of intramyocardial vessel, were described by Wearn *et al.* [4]. They showed for the first time direct histologic and gross evidence of the myocardial sinusoidal plexus with its arteriosinusoidal, luminal–sinusoidal, and arterioluminal com-

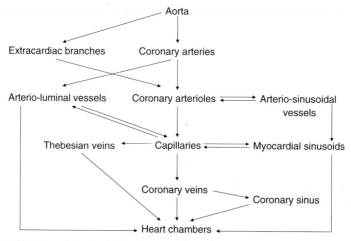

Figure 4.1 Blood supply to the ischemic myocardium after occlusion. These accessory pathways may also be called coronary collateral circulation.

ponents. It was believed that, before reaching the heart chambers, these thin-walled channels anastomosed with adjacent sinusoidal vessels and with capillaries that lie in close contact with muscle fibers in order to support oxygen exchange [1]. Although this was only speculated for the human heart, in the sponge-like reptilian heart these sinusoidal vessels do allow the myocardium to be perfused directly from the ventricular chambers [5] – from which the idea of transmyocardial revascularization of the severely ischemic myocardium was born.

Effect of the laser source on myocardial tissue

Principles

Laser is an acronym for "light amplification by stimulated emission of radiation." A laser works by bombarding molecules in a medium with an outside energy source (light, electricity, etc.). This bombardment brings the orbital electrons of these molecules to a higher level of excitation, from which they drop back to the original orbit and, in the process, emit a photon. For a given molecule and incoming energy, the energy of the emitted photon is fixed. The photon oscillates between two reflective mirrors placed in the laser cavity, hitting numerous other molecules and exciting their electrons. This amplification process continues until photons fill the cavity. Finally, one of the mirrors is removed from the path of the photons, releasing the photons to form a laser beam. If all molecules in the laser cavity are identical, the energy of the photons making up the laser beam is identical. This type of monochromaticity imparts a high degree of coherence, giving the laser beam its power [6].

Effect of laser wavelength and pulse parameters

Photonic vibrations (wavelength and frequency) determine the "color" and energy of the laser radiation. The wavelength and frequency are inversely proportional; in other words, photons with more energy vibrate faster and have a shorter wavelength, whereas less energetic photons have lower frequency and a longer wavelength. If the wavelength of the photon is 400–700 nm, it becomes visible. Any light with a wavelength shorter than 400 nm is referred to as ultraviolet (UV). By contrast, any light with a wavelength longer than 700 nm is called infrared (IR). The relationship between wavelength of the laser photons and the natural vibrational frequency of the target tissue molecules determines how strongly laser radiation is absorbed and/or scattered in the irradiated media. The excimer laser (xenon-chloride, XeCl) is an example of a UV laser that is capable of breaking the dipeptide bonds (molecular dissociation) in the target tissue. However, holmium:yttrium-aluminum-garnet (Ho:YAG) and carbon dioxide (CO_2) lasers are examples of IR lasers that interact with the tissue by heating water molecules (thermal effect). Because myocardial tissue is made up by water and protein, it is possible to conduct TMR using excimer, Ho:YAG, or CO_2 lasers.

The energy of the photons determines the forward ablation speed of the laser beam that carries the photons. In other words, the more energetic photons will penetrate target tissue deeper and remove larger chunks of material that lies in the path of the laser beam. In regard to TMR, this means that the high-energy CO_2 laser (20–60 J/pulse) can perforate myocardium with a single shot. Ho:YAG and XeCl lasers operate at low energy levels (1 J and 250 mJ/pulse) and require 10–20 pulses (Ho:YAG) or more than 40 pulses (XeCl) to create a single transmyocardial channel. The extent of collateral damage is determined by the peak power generated by the laser photons inside the target tissue. Peak power is the pulse energy divided by pulse duration. The CO_2 laser generates 20–60 J of energy by pulse over a period of 10–100 ms, corresponding to peak energy levels of 800–1000 W. By contrast, the Ho:YAG laser, which generates a much lower

Table 4.1 Histologic damage in cardiovascular tissue during transmyocardial laser revascularization (TMR) with three laser modalities. From Kadipasaoglu *et al.* [9] with permission.

Variables	CO_2	Ho:YAG	XeCl
Channel diameter (mm)	1.0	0.6	0.6
Unilateral damage (mm)*	0.52 ± 0.25	1.84 ± 0.67	0.74 ± 0.18
Volumetric damage (cm³)*†	1.49 ± 1.03	8.46 ± 5.35	1.87 ± 0.72

CO_2, carbon dioxide laser; Ho:YAG, holmium:yttrium-aluminum-garnet laser; XeCl, xenon-chloride laser.

* Mean ± standard deviation.

† For 30 channels made in 2-cm thick porcine myocardium, excluding channel volume.

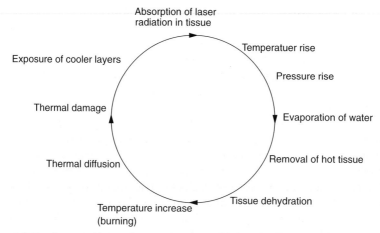

Figure 4.2 Events caused by continuous-wave laser ablation of soft tissue. From Jansen *et al.* [8] with permission.

energy of approximately 1 J/pulse, delivers it in such short duration (250 μs) that the peak developed power is 10-fold that of the CO_2 laser. The peak power of the XeCl laser is yet another order of magnitude higher because of the extremely short duration of the pulse (250 ns) [6,7]. Table 4.1 summarizes the histologic damage in porcine cardiovascular tissue during TMR with the three laser modalities discussed above.

Immediate effects

In vitro
When laser radiation is absorbed by water in myocardial tissue, the tissue rapidly heats to a temperature of 100–150°C. After energy conversion causes vaporization, local dehydration of the tissue occurs, and the temperature increases to 350–450°C, which causes tissue carbonization and ablation. The exposure of deep, cooler tissues to the continuing ablation process results in the creation of myocardial channels (Fig. 4.2) [8]. The channel depth is dependent on the laser energy delivered to the tissue and increases logarithmically with time. With a CO_2 laser, a pulse duration of 20 ms is sufficient to traverse 20 mm of myocardial tissue with a single shot under *in vitro* experimental conditions. Birefringence microscopy has shown that increasing the pulse duration contributes to increased thermal damage in the tissue adjacent to the channel. Moreover, thermally altered tissue damage and tissue tearing was found to be more pronounced parallel to the myofibrils as compared with the damage perpendicular to the myofibrils. In addition, when the heart is filled with water or blood in *in vitro* conditions, these fluids stop the laser beam once the myocardial wall is entirely traversed [8].

In vivo

Macroscopic

We assessed tissue damage of three different types of lasers in an experimental pig model [9]. After treatment with a Ho:YAG laser at a pulse energy of 2 J, pulse duration 250×10^{-3}, and a pulse frequency of $10 \, s^{-1}$, the entry points of the laser shots on the epicardial surface were demarcated by a thin circle of hemorrhage surrounded by a white, concentric circular zone showing the thermal effects of laser irradiation. The appearance of the endocardial exit points of the laser shots were similar to the entry points on the epicardial surface. Irregular, transmural channels measuring up to 2 mm were surrounded by an extensive area of discoloration (Fig. 4.3). Although the hearts treated with the XeCl laser showed generally similar changes, epicardial laser entry spots were smaller in diameter,

(a)

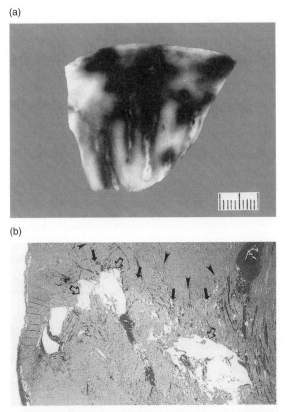

(b)

Figure 4.3 Gross and histologic appearance of myocardial tissue after treatment with a Ho:YAG laser. The laser was operated at a pulse energy of 2 J, a pulse duration of 250×10^{-3} s, and a pulse frequency of $10 \, s^{-1}$. (a) Longitudinal section with transmural appearance of the track; note the zigzag path of the track. (b) Photomicrograph of a midmural section. The open arrows point to the laser channels; the closed arrows point to the borders of the zone of irreversible coagulation damage; the arrowheads point to the zone of reversible damage (with an admixture of changes). (Hematoxylin and eosin stain; original magnification, ×40.) From Kadipasaoglu *et al.* [9] with permission.

and the width of the irregular transmyocardial laser channels was much narrower than that of the channels in the hearts of animals treated with the Ho:YAG laser (Fig. 4.4). The epicardial (entry) and endocardial (exit) spots of the CO_2 laser channels were surrounded by a 1-mm diameter concentric circle of hemorrhagic tissue. On longitudinal sections, the vicinity of straight laser channels traversing the myocardium was also surrounded by this circle of collateral damage (Fig. 4.5) [9].

Microscopic
For all lasers, immediate light microscopic evaluation of the longitudinal and transverse myocardial sections showed open elliptical channels surrounded by four concentric zones of vaporization, carbonization, fixation, and transition in

(a)

(b)

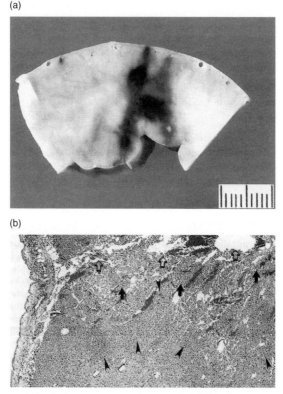

Figure 4.4 Gross and histologic appearance of myocardial tissue after treatment with an XeCl. The laser was operated at a pulse energy of 0.035 J, a pulse duration of 20×10^{-9} s, and a pulse frequency of 30 s^{-1}. (a) Transmural cross-section of an irregular channel. (b) Photomicrograph of a subepicardial section. The open arrows point to the laser channels; the closed arrows point to the borders of the zone of irreversible coagulation damage; and arrowheads show the zone of reversible damage (with an admixture of changes). (Hematoxylin and eosin stain; original magnification, ×40.) From Kadipasaoglu *et al.* [9] with permission.

(a)

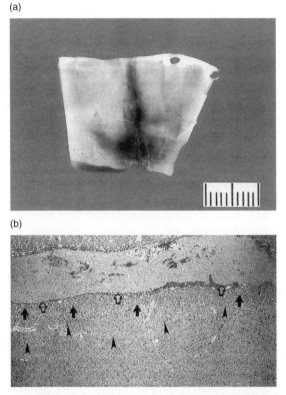

(b)

Figure 4.5 Gross and histologic appearance of myocardial tissue after treatment with a CO_2 laser. The laser was operated at a pulse energy of 20 J and a pulse duration of 19×10^{-3} s. (a) Transmural cross-section. (b) Photomicrograph of a midmural section. Open arrows point to laser channels; closed arrows show the borders of the zone of coagulation damage; and arrowheads point to the zone of reversible damage (with an admixture of changes). (Hematoxylin and eosin stain; original magnification, ×40.) From Kadipasaoglu *et al*. [9] with permission.

the adjacent myocardial tissue. The long axes of those elliptical channels were parallel to the muscle fiber planes, and their lumens were filled with coagulated proteins, strands of fibrin, erythrocytes, and necrotic debris (Figs 4.3–4.5). A zone of thermal damage or coagulation, which was larger in the direction of the muscle fibers, surrounded this ablated lumen [9,10]. In this region, the cardiac myocyte morphology was dense. Eosinophilic cytoplasm was present, and myocytes typically contained hypercontraction bands, pyknotic to absent nuclei. The next zone had structural changes. Within scattered myocytes were coagulation necrosis, vacuolar changes, contraction band changes, and wavy fiber changes. This perimeter zone was further accentuated by extravasated erythrocytes in the interstitial space that corresponded to the hemorrhagic outer circles in the gross sections. The zone of structural damage blended into the histologically normal tissue [9,11].

The extent of the thermal and acoustic damage varied among the different lasers. In an *in vitro* study, the erbium:YAG (Er:YAG) channel was reported to have the least thermal damage when the created channels were compared with the channels created by Ho:YAG and CO_2 lasers [10]. The Er:YAG is an infrared laser like the Ho:YAG and CO_2 lasers. It interacts with water, but its water absorption peak is higher than that of the Ho:YAG laser. Therefore, it scatters less and creates less collateral damage. However, in other *in vitro* studies, the tissue damage caused by a CO_2 laser was found to be considerably less than that caused by the XeCl and Ho:YAG lasers [9,12]. The XeCl and Ho:YAG lasers have shorter pulse durations than the CO_2 laser, and they cause more myocardial trauma, possibly because of their higher peak powers. Moreover, these low-energy, short-pulse Ho:YAG and XeCl lasers cause only slight forward ablation, thus requiring several pulses to create a single channel. A number of these pulses may cause arrhythmias when they coincide with the T wave [13]. To minimize arrhythmias after treatment, electrocardiogram-triggered activation was proposed [9].

Perfusion has also been looked at microscopically. In their acute ischemic model, Kohmoto *et al.* [11] demonstrated histologically that blood can penetrate into the myocardial wall directly through the channels created by the Ho:YAG laser; however, this slightly increased blood flow was not enough to perfuse ischemic areas and maintain viability. After TMR treatment with a CO_2 laser in another experimental study, there was less perfusion in the regions proximal (1–2 mm) and distal to channels (>3 mm) than before treatment [14]. Similarly, Mueller *et al.* [15] also suggested that TMR might first cause low flow and local ischemia following a transient drop of ejection fraction and hypokinesis, which could reverse within 30 minutes.

Effects at 1–24 hours

Studies of the three lasers typically used for TMR show similar findings. In one experimental study, laser channels created with a XeCl laser were shown to be open 1 hour after treatment [16]. The channel diameter and tissue damage increased with the catheter diameter and pulse frequency. In an autopsy study of TMR with a CO_2 laser, laser channels were identified to be open on myocardial section. However, histologic examination showed a 1- to 2-mm broad rim of carbonization, early myofibrillary degeneration, and edema around the channels in the autopsy of a patient who died 2 hours after being treated with a CO_2 laser. Clotting of the channels was detected near the epicardial surface, but no fibrin thrombi were reported. There were also direct communications between some of the channels, the native myocardial vessels, and the ventricular cavity, which suggests that early channel patency does not correlate with the decline of the left ventricular function [17].

In another experimental, comparative study of the CO_2 and Ho:YAG lasers, all elliptically shaped laser channels were identifiable 6–24 hours after treatment [12]. No differences in channel characteristics were seen among the animals. For both lasers, the histologic appearance of the surrounding tissue was consistent with thermal tissue necrosis and thermal-acoustic damage, showing zones of contraction band necrosis, widening of the perivascular interstitium, and varying degrees of fascicular separation. The channels also contained fresh thrombus, which suggested that there was not substantial flow through these acute channels. In some sections, interstitial blood could be identified extending from the channel site. The lumen size and the area of thermal damage of the CO_2 laser channels were both smaller than that of the Ho:YAG laser [12]. At autopsy of a patient who died in the early postoperative period (24 hours), Sigel *et al.* [18] found that the CO_2 laser channels were not patent and were filled with protein, blood, and inflammatory cells and that there was restricted collateral damage to the adjacent myocardium. This result is consistent with previously mentioned reports and does not support the theory of improved myocardial perfusion from the left ventricle by means of laser channels [19].

Effects at 3–7 days

The histopathologic examination of the heart of a patient who died on postoperative day 3, reported by Gasler *et al.* [20], showed that the CO_2 laser channels were sealed with fibrinous precipitations both at the epicardium and endocardium. In the epicardium, the fatty tissue adjacent to the channel entry was necrotic and infiltrated by granulocytes, erythrocytes, thrombocytes, and red cells. The adjacent fatty tissue was necrotic and densely infiltrated by granulocytes and some erythrocytes. The channels were not patent, and they were filled with a fibrinous network containing granulocytes and some erythrocytes. Endothelial and proliferating cells were not present in the channels. The myocardial defects were characterized by altered muscle tissue. A thin layer of myocytic detritus was found contiguous to the defects; there was a border zone of coagulation necrosis, which was infiltrated by granulocytes. The adjacent zone in the myocardium had prominently enlarged cardiomyocytes with fibrillar cytoplasmic degenerations and an adjoining layer of typical contraction band necrosis. The myocardium was neither extensively infiltrated by erythrocytes, nor was there positive Prussian blue iron staining of adjacent laser-created channels [20].

Similarly, in their experimental study in pigs, Chu *et al.* [21] could not demonstrate a patent channel 1 week after CO_2 laser treatment or after needle puncture. Rather, laser channels were seen as fibrous tracts containing fibroblasts and collagen with occasional small blood vessels. The fibrous tracts were narrower than the original laser beam diameter, were surrounded by granulation tissue and damaged myocardium, and included infiltrating lymphocytes and macrophages, a similar inflammatory process as that seen in normal tissue healing. As evidence of inflammation-mediated angiogenic response, there were numerous small vascular structures (<10 µm in diameter with vascular endothelial growth factor [VEGF]-stained endothelium) in the area of inflammation. An increase in vascular density was also reported. Although the inflammatory changes were similar to those that occur after needle puncture, the inflammatory response created by laser injury was greater [21].

Effects at 10 days to 2 weeks

Specimens taken by various investigators at human autopsies have not shown patent channels at 10 days to 2 weeks. In one specimen, the channels were filled with fibroblasts, macrophages, lymphocytes, and other chronic inflammatory cells. The thermal damage zone, however, was reduced [18]. Similar results were seen in an autopsy specimen from a patient treated with the Ho:YAG laser [22]. In addition, those histologic changes were also associated with vascularization of granulation tissue. Burkhoff *et al.* [22] called the outcome of these changes "channel remnants." Animal experiments have also shown that channel remnants were lined with endothelium and surrounded by capillary networks [23,24].

Effects at 3–4 weeks

No evidence of channel patency between the left ventricle and myocardium has been reported at 1 month in several experimental studies [25–27]. The channels consisted of scar tissue, which was composed of numerous thickened collagen fibers and arteriolar structures, and there was evidence of neovascularization [25–27]. In one of these studies, the vascular density and arteriolar structures in granulation tissue in the non-treated, control group were half that of the group treated with a Ho:YAG laser [28]. VEGF and adenovirus injections stimulated more myocardial inflammation but no additional angiogenesis at 1 month [27]. In an experimental dose–response study, histologic examination of myocardial tissue lased with the excimer laser showed similar findings, including an inflammatory response and a high degree of neovascularization in the loose connective tissue surrounding the channels [29]. Semiquantitative and quantitative analysis of technetium-99m-sestamibi (^{99m}Tc-sestamibi) perfusion scans showed significant ($P < 0.004$) improvement in stress-induced ischemia 4 weeks after 50-channel TMR compared with scans obtained immediately before lasing. Moreover, 25- and 10-channel TMR did not demonstrate as significant an improvement in stress-induced ischemia as that obtained after 50-channel TMR [29]. In another model, improved perfusion in ischemic areas following Ho:YAG laser treatment was shown by high-spatial-resolution cine magnetic resonance imaging (MRI) [30]. Histologic findings of human autopsy specimens at 3 and 4 weeks were consistent with the animal experiments [18,31].

Effects at 4–8 weeks

Elliptical scars, representing the scarred channel entry points, were identified on the endocardial surface by Fisher *et al.* [12] at 4–8 weeks. These entry sites were not patent in any of the experimental cases at 6 weeks. The abundant neovascularization present within the scar at 2–3 weeks decreased at 6 weeks. The degree of vascularization within the scar tissue that replaced the channel lumen was highly variable and included capillaries and arterioles. According to Fisher *et al.*:

> "As with the acute studies, the dimensions of the chronic laser channel remnant did not vary significantly throughout the area of the left ventricular wall with either laser. The area of channel remnant, which was dramatically reduced at 2 to 3 weeks as compared with the original area of thermal damage (the area of involvement was generally larger for Ho:YAG than for the CO_2 laser), was reduced even further at 6 weeks so that the majority of the channels were entirely replaced with vascular fibrous tissue consistent with completed scar. The area of involvement became the same for the 2 lasers at 6 weeks. The appearance of laser channels at these time points were, therefore, consistent with an evolving, richly vascular cicatricial process." [12]

In a study comparing the chronic effects of three laser sources, all channels became occluded by scar within 6 weeks [10]. The Er:YAG laser produced minimal acute thermal damage, which corresponded to smaller scars. The pulsed Ho:YAG laser caused stronger tissue tearing than continuous wave CO_2 irradiation. With all lasers, the volume density of intramyocardial vessels increased around the scar tissue 6 weeks after treatment. According to Genyk *et al.* [10], "Rapid channel occlusion suggests that rather than revascularization, subsidiary physiologic tissue effects elicited by the thermal, oxidative, or mechanical action of the laser impact may contribute to the beneficial clinical effects of TMR."

In 1995, Horvath *et al.* [32] described patent laser channels in a sheep model 30 days after laser treatment. Histologic analysis of the lased (XeCl) and mechanically revascularized ischemic areas using immunohistochemical methods showed less scar development in lased than in non-lased regions. In addition, only laser-treated ischemic tissue showed a significant increase in the number of blood vessels (neovascularization) [33]. In response to these findings, Beranek [34] stated that even though the laser channels are obstructed by damaged cardiomyocytes and impermeable to red cells, they might have been permeable to interstitial fluid and permitted the washout of lactate and the supply of glucose in the ischemic myocardium, which is dependent on anaerobic glycolysis for its survival. This theory also agrees with the possibility that a limited amount of blood may have penetrated into the channels and that blood might be able to pass freely through the channels after the hyalinized cardiomyocytes are fragmented.

Effects at 8–12 weeks

In an experimental study, comparing the additive effect of fibroblast growth factor (bFGF) to TMR, Yamamoto *et al.* [35] found that granulation tissue with significant vascular structures infiltrated all TMR channels at 8 weeks, independent of whether they did or did not have bFGF. Accordingly, the channel remnant areas were significantly larger in the bFGF group than in the TMR alone group. This difference likely reflects increased fibroblast proliferation induced by the growth factor. In both cases in this study, many of the smooth muscle and endothelial cells within the remnants incorporated 5-bromo-2'-deoxyuridine (BrdU), which indicated actively growing vessels. Thus, active vascular growth was likely completed before the 2-month sacrifice. According to Yamamoto *et al.* [35]:

> "In both TMLR and TMLR+bFGF groups, vascular density and cellular proliferation were markedly increased in the normal myocardium surrounding the channel remnants when compared to the control group. However, addition of bFGF to the channels was associated with evidence of vascular proliferation in much larger arteries and at greater distances from the channel remnants. It is rare to see vessels of this size deep in the myocardium; furthermore, we have never observed this degree of BrdU incorporation in an artery of this size in control ischemic hearts or even following TMLR." [35]

Yamamoto *et al.* also observed other effects of bFGF. In some channels, they found extensive fibrosis and there was unorganized vascular proliferation (Fig. 4.6a,b). In addition, they saw highly organized stimulation of conduit vessel growth (Fig. 4.6c,d). To make a quantitative comparison, they determined vascular density and proliferating vascular cell density in different areas of each heart. "Vascular density in the normal myocardium immediately surrounding

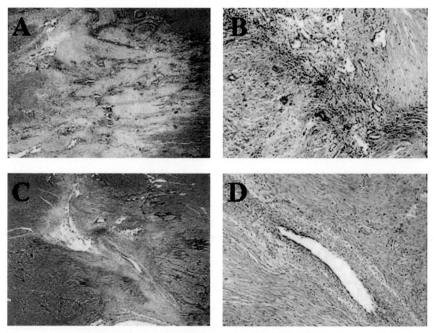

Figure 4.6 Histologic appearance of channel remnants 2 months after treatment in patients who had transmyocardial laser revascularization and basic fibroblast growth. (a,b) Extensive fibrosis and intense, unorganized vascular proliferation. (c,d) Large mature vessels observed traversing the channel remnant with much less unorganized angiogenesis. Trichrome stained samples; original magnification ×40 in (a), ×100 in (b), 20× in (c), and ×200 in (d). From Yamamoto *et al.* [35] with permission.

(a)

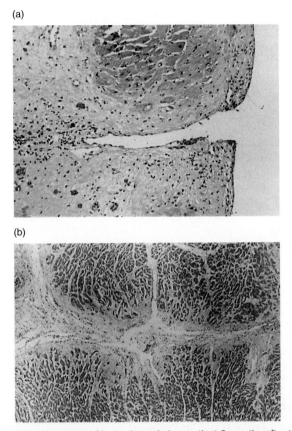

(b)

Figure 4.7 Histologic appearance of laser channels in a patient 3 months after treatment. (a) Channel connecting to the endocardium. (Hematoxylin and eosin stain; original magnification ×100.) (b) Channel connecting to intramyocardial vasculature. (Hematoxylin and eosin stain; original magnification ×40.) From Cooley *et al.* [37] with permission.

the TMLR channel remnants and in the region neighboring the channel remnants were comparable in the TMLR and TMLR+bFGF groups." [35]

In another postmortem study of a patient treated by a XeCl laser performed at week 12, van der Sloot *et al.* [36] showed that all channels were closed. However, as in the animal studies, angiogenesis was present in the fibrotic channels and the adjacent myocardial tissue. Only one human postmortem histologic study revealed anatomic evidence of patent laser channels, which were created with the CO_2 laser (Fig. 4.7) [37]. Although reactive fibrous scar tissue caused narrowing of the original laser tract, the channels had endothelialized and they contained red blood cells, which suggested that they were still patent.

Effects at 5–6 months

Hughes *et al.* [7] compared the 6-month effects of three different lasers (CO_2, Ho:YAG, and XeCl) in ischemic pig hearts. Histologic staining of the channel remnants revealed hypocellular regions filled with connective tissue, and no patent channels were seen in any of the study groups. Endogenous endothelial alkaline phosphatase staining demonstrated numerous blood vessels and increased vascular density in the vicinity of CO_2 and Ho:YAG channel remnants compared with those areas of XeCl lased and non-lased regions. Moreover, vascular density was found to be greater in Ho:YAG than in CO_2 treated myocardium. Positron emission tomography (PET) scans showed increased myocardial blood flow to the regions lased by CO_2 and Ho:YAG lasers when compared with pretreatment flow ($P < 0.002$ and $P < 0.001$, respectively). However, the change was not significant after XeCl laser treatment [7].

Gassler *et al.* [20] did not report any open laser channels 5 months after laser treatment. In their patient, the channels were healed with scar tissue, which was associated with an extensive capillary network. They also found some connections between endothelialized structures of the laser channels and left ventricular cavity.

Effects at 9 months

In two different autopsies performed 9 months after TMR with a CO_2 laser, gross inspection of the myocardium did not show any patent channels within the lased regions [38,39]. Microscopic evaluation showed channel remnants and minimal perichannel scarring. Multiple vessels containing red blood cells were shown within and adjacent to the channel remnants. In addition, capillary vascular density analysis of the lased areas revealed a significantly higher vessel count than non-lased areas ($P < 0.001$) [39].

Conclusions

As can be inferred from this review, controversy remains regarding the mechanism and efficacy of TMR. Only a new prospective, randomized, multicenter trial could resolve the controversy. The trial should be conducted on a sufficiently large number of sole-therapy patients and by using an advanced diagnostic technique such as gaited PET or perfusion MRI. One-to-one comparisons of cardiac perfusion between baseline and 12 months or more follow-up should be performed by blinded experts at a core facility.

Acknowledgments

The authors would like to thank Richard Jude and Marianne Mallia-Hughes, ELS, of the Texas Heart Institute's Department of Scientific Publications for their editorial assistance in preparing this chapter.

References

1 Cohen, MV. Morphologic considerations of the coronary collateral circulation in man. In: Cohen MV (ed.) *Coronary Collaterals: Clinical and Experimental Observations*. Mount Kisco, New York: Futura Publishing Co., 1985 : 1–79.

2 Vieussens R. *Nouvelles Découvertes sur le Coeur, Expliquées dans une Lettre Ecrite a Monsieur Boudin, Conseiller d'Etat, Premier Medicin de Monseigneur*. Paris: Laurent d'Houry, 1706.

3 Leibowitz JO. *The History of Coronary Heart Disease*. University of California Press, Berkeley, 1970.

4 Wearn JT, Mettier SR, Klumpp TG, Zschiesche LJ. The nature of the vascular communications between the coronary arteries and the chambers of the heart. *Am Heart J* 1933;**9**: 143–64.

5 Kohmoto T, Argenziano M, Yamamoto N, *et al*. Assessment of transmyocardial perfusion in alligator hearts. *Circulation* 1997;**95**:1585–91.

6 Kadipasaoglu KA, Frazier OH. Transmyocardial laser revascularization: effect of laser parameters on tissue ablation and cardiac perfusion. *Semin Thorac Cardiovasc Surg* 1999;**11**:4–11.

7 Hughes GC, Kypson AP, Annex BH, *et al*. Induction of angiogenesis after TMR: a comparison of holmium:YAG, CO_2, and excimer lasers. *Ann Thorac Surg* 2000;**70**:504–9.

8 Jansen ED, Frenz M, Kadipasaoglu KA, *et al*. Laser–tissue interaction during transmyocardial laser revascularization. *Ann Thorac Surg* 1997;**63**:640–67.

9 Kadipasaoglu KA, Sartori M, Masai T, *et al*. Intraoperative arrhythmias and tissue damage during transmyocardial laser revascularization. *Ann Thorac Surg* 1999;**67**:423–31.

10 Genyk IA, Frenz M, Ott B, *et al*. Acute and chronic effects of transmyocardial laser revascularization in the nonischemic pig myocardium by using three laser systems. *Lasers Surg Med* 2000;**27**:438–50.

11 Kohmoto T, Fisher PE, Gu A, *et al*. Does blood flow through holmium:YAG transmyocardial laser channels? *Ann Thorac Surg* 1996;**61**:861–8.

12 Fisher PE, Khomoto T, DeRosa CM, *et al*. Histologic analysis of transmyocardial channels: comparison of CO_2 and holmium:YAG lasers. *Ann Thorac Surg* 1997;**64**:466–72.

13 Frazier OH, Tuzun E, Kadipasaoglu K. Management of refractory angina not amenable to conventional therapy. In: Wheatley DJ. (ed) *Surgery of Coronary Artery Disease*, 2nd edn. London: Arnold, 2003: 382–93.

14 Hattan N, Ban K, Tanaka E, *et al*. Transmyocardial revascularization aggravates myocardial ischemia around the channels in the immediate phase. *Am J Physiol Heart Circ Physiol* 2000;**279**:H1392–6.

15 Mueller XM, Tevaearai H, Genton CY, Bettex D, von Segesser LK. Laser transmyocardial revascularization: a potential risk in an acute situation? *Swiss Surg* 2000;**6**:65–8.

16 Shehada RE, Papaioannou T, Mansour HN, Grundfest WS. Excimer laser (308 nm) based transmyocardial laser revascularization: effects of the lasing parameters on myocardial histology. *Lasers Surg Med* 2001;**29**:85–91.

17 Lutter G, Schwarzkopf J, Lutz C, Martin J, Beyersdorf F. Histologic findings of transmyocardial laser channels after two hours. *Ann Thorac Surg* 1998;**65**:1437–9.

18 Sigel JE, Abramovich CM, Lytle BW, Ratliff NB. Transmyocardial laser revascularization: three sequential autopsy cases. *J Thorac Cardiovasc Surg* 1998;**115**:1381–5.

19 Cherian SM, Bobryshev YV, Liang H, *et al*. Ultrastructural and immunohistochemical analysis of early myocardial changes following transmyocardial laser revascularization. *J Cardiol Surg* 2000;**15**:341–6.

20 Gassler N, Wintzer HO, Stubbe HM, Wullbrand A, Helmchen U. Transmyocardial laser revascularization: histological features in human nonresponder myocardium. *Circulation* 1997;**95**:371–5.

21 Chu VF, Giaid A, Kuang JQ, *et al*. Angiogenesis in transmyocardial revascularization: comparison of laser versus mechanical punctures. *Ann Thorac Surg* 1999;**68**:301–7.

22 Burkhoff D, Fulton R, Wharton K, Billingham ME, Robbins R. Myocardial perfusion through naturally occurring subendocardial channels. *J Thorac Cardiovasc Surg* 1997;**114**:497–9.

23 Li W, Tanaka K, Chiba Y, *et al.* Role of MMPs and plasminogen activators in angiogenesis after transmyocardial laser revascularization in dogs. *Am J Physiol Heart Circ Physiol* 2003;**284**:H23–30.

24 Kohmoto T, Fisher PE, Gu A, *et al.* Physiology, histology, and 2-week morphology of acute transmyocardial channels made with a CO_2 laser. *Ann Thorac Surg* 1997;**63**:1275–83.

25 Mueller XM, Tevaearai HT, Chaubert P, Genton CY, von Segesser LK. Does laser injury induce a different neovascularisation pattern from mechanical or ischaemic injuries? *Heart* 2001;**85**:697–701.

26 Mack CA, Magovern CJ, Hahn RT, *et al.* Channel patency and neovascularization after transmyocardial revascularization using an excimer laser: results and comparisons to non-lased channels. *Circulation* 1997;**96**(Suppl 2):65–9.

27 Fleischer KJ, Goldschmidt-Clermont PJ, Fonger JD, *et al.* One-month histologic response of transmyocardial laser channels with molecular intervention. *Ann Thorac Surg* 1996;**62**:1051–8.

28 Mueller XM, Tevaearai HT, Genton CY, Chaubert P, von Segesser LK. Are there vascular density gradients along myocardial laser channels? *Ann Thorac Surg* 1999;**68**:125–9.

29 Hamawy AH, Lee LY, Samy SA, *et al.* Transmyocardial laser revascularization dose response: enhanced perfusion in a porcine ischemia model as a function of channel density. *Ann Thorac Surg* 2001;**72**:817–22.

30 Nahrendorf M, Hiller KH, Theisen D, *et al.* Effect of transmyocardial laser revascularization on myocardial perfusion and left ventricular remodeling after myocardial infarction in rats. *Radiology* 2002;**225**:487–93.

31 Burkhoff D, Fisher PE, Apfelbaum M, *et al.* Histologic appearance of transmyocardial laser channels after 4 1/2 weeks. *Ann Thorac Surg* 1996;**61**:1532–4.

32 Horvath KA, Smith WJ, Laurence RG, *et al.* Recovery and viability of an acute myocardial infarct after transmyocardial laser revascularization. *J Am Coll Cardiol* 1995;**25**:258–63.

33 Horvath KA, Belkind N, Wu I, *et al.* Functional comparison of transmyocardial revascularization by mechanical and laser means. *Ann Thorac Surg* 2001;**72**:1997–2002.

34 Beranek JT. Pseudovascular tubes obscure transmyocardial revascularization. *Ann Thorac Surg* 1997;**63**:597–8.

35 Yamamoto N, Kohmoto T, Roethy W, *et al.* Histologic evidence that basic fibroblast growth factor enhances the angiogenic effects of transmyocardial laser revascularization. *Basic Res Cardiol* 2000;**95**:55–63.

36 van der Sloot JA, Huikeshoven M, van der Wal AC, *et al.* Angiogenesis three months after clinical transmyocardial laser revascularization using an excimer laser. *Lasers Surg Med* 2001;**29**:369–73.

37 Cooley DA, Frazier OH, Kadipasaoglu KA, *et al.* Transmyocardial laser revascularization: anatomic evidence of long-term channel patency. *Tex Heart Inst J* 1994;**21**:220–4.

38 Summers JH, Henry AC 3, Roberts WC. Cardiac observations late after operative transmyocardial laser "revascularization." *Am J Cardiol* 1999;**84**:489–90.

39 Domkowski PW, Biswas SS, Steenbergen C, Lowe JE. Histological evidence of angiogenesis 9 months after transmyocardial laser revascularization. *Circulation* 2001;**103**:469–71.

CHAPTER 5

Animal models of acute and chronic coronary ischemia: effects of TMR on perfusion and left ventricular function

G Chad Hughes and James E Lowe

Introduction

Since its description, transmyocardial laser revascularization (TMR) has been tested extensively in numerous animal experiments before proceeding to clinical application [1]. This chapter outlines the various ischemic animal models utilized to date in preclinical studies of TMR and details their results regarding changes in myocardial perfusion and function after the procedure. Data on histologic findings as well as purely morphologic studies without functional endpoints are not addressed but are covered elsewhere in this textbook. In addition, studies combining the use of TMR with various pro-angiogenic growth factors are not examined as the purpose of the chapter is to examine the effects of TMR alone.

Acute myocardial ischemia models

TMR is generally performed in patients with chronic effort-induced myocardial ischemia, and is, in fact, contraindicated in patients with acute coronary syndromes [2]. Thus, studies of acute ischemia have limited clinical applicability. However, these models have been very useful in early studies examining the mechanism of action of TMR and investigation into whether the laser channels can acutely increase regional perfusion [3]. Several different species have been used in acute ischemia or infarct models including rats, dogs, sheep, and pigs. Each of these is outlined below.

Rat models

These models have generally utilized ligation of the left coronary artery in rats. Because rats have a limited native collateral circulation [4], this produces myocardial infarction in the distribution of the left coronary artery. One disadvantage of the rat model is a high mortality rate (up to 50%) following coronary ligation, as well as significant variability in infarct size [5]. In addition, direct measurement of regional myocardial blood flow and function is more difficult than in larger animal models. As a consequence, no study to date has assessed perfusion or function pre-TMR and post-TMR in the rat model. Rather, studies have used indirect markers such as infarct size as a surrogate for regional flow. The inherent variability in infarct size with this model, however, introduces the possibility of type I error (i.e., finding a significant difference between groups when one does not actually exist) unless large numbers of animals are randomized into treatment and control groups.

Few rat studies of acute ischemia with functional endpoints have been published. All involve the creation of TMR channels in non-ischemic myocardium followed by an acute ischemic challenge some time later and assess the ability of TMR to provide myocardial protection in this setting. Guo et al. [6] ligated the left coronary artery of rats immediately followed by the creation of transmural channels using an neodymium:yttrium-aluminium-garnet (Nd:YAG) laser. Laser treated rats had reduced myocardial infarct (MI) size and enzyme leakage, and improved left ventricular function compared with controls. Whittaker et al. [7] created transmural holmium:YAG and needle channels in the left ventricle of rats. Two months later, the left coronary artery was occluded for 90 minutes followed by 4.5 hours of reperfusion. Findings included a decrease in infarct size in treated animals compared with sham operated controls. A follow-up study [8] from this same group using a similar coronary occlusion protocol investigated the effects of TMR channels created using a frequency-tripled Nd:YAG laser at high- and low-pulse energy levels. Two to 5 months after TMR, the left coronary artery was occluded for 90 minutes as in the prior study. Infarct size was significantly less in those animals treated using the high-pulse energy setting.

Canine models

These models have typically involved ligation of one or more coronary arteries either prior to or after TMR was performed. Aside from the limitations of acute models of ischemia for the study of TMR noted above, a drawback of the canine model is the variable and often substantial collateral circulation network. These preformed collaterals are capable of providing up to 40% of normal flow to the perfusion bed of an acutely occluded epicardial coronary artery [4]. Regardless, much of the early work investigating TMR was performed using the canine model. In their sentinel report in 1981, Mirhoseini and Cayton [9] described the use of a 400-W CO_2 laser to create 20–30 transmural channels in the left ventricle of dogs either before or shortly after occlusion of the left anterior descending (LAD) coronary artery. TMR appeared to provide a protective effect, as there was a significant reduction in mortality in animals treated with TMR either pre- or post-ligation compared with untreated controls. Similar results were reported by others [10,11]. In none of these studies was regional myocardial blood flow or function directly measured before or after TMR.

Yano et al. [12] performed endocardial holmium:YAG TMR to create non-transmural channels prior to 90 minutes of LAD occlusion. Sonomicrometers and echocardiography were used to assess regional contractility in lased and non-lased dogs. Findings included improved regional contractility in the lased animals during a 4-hour reperfusion period, although mortality was higher in the lased group. Landreneau et al. [13] occluded the LAD of dogs after CO_2 laser

TMR of the anterior wall of the left ventricle. Compared with controls, there was no improvement in regional myocardial blood flow as measured using radioactive microspheres or function by sonomicrometric analysis in TMR treated animals following LAD occlusion. Similarly, Whittaker *et al.* [14] found no improvement in regional myocardial blood flow or function (Fig. 5.1) and no difference in infarct size in dogs undergoing holmium:YAG TMR 30 minutes after ligation of the LAD versus untreated controls. Likewise, no evidence for transmyocardial blood flow via TMR channels in the distribution of a ligated LAD was seen using isolated, perfused canine heart models [15,16]. Further, Kadipasaoglu *et al.* [17] have demonstrated no acute improvement in regional myocardial function when TMR with a high power CO_2 laser is performed prior to LAD ligation in dogs. However, regional function was improved over untreated controls 3 months post-ligation.

Ovine models

As in the rat and canine models, the sheep acute ischemia models used to investigate TMR have generally involved coronary occlusion. Unlike dogs, however, sheep appear to have fewer pre-existing coronary collaterals, and thus a larger area of MI results [18]. Horvath *et al.* [18] investigated the effects of CO_2 laser TMR on regional function early and late after LAD ligation in sheep. They found a slight but significant improvement in regional function during a 3-hour period after LAD ligation in TMR treated sheep versus controls. This preservation in regional function was even greater 30 days postoperatively in the TMR treated animals. The observed acute improvement in regional function after TMR in this study contrasts with other acute ischemic sheep studies. Eckstein *et al.* [19,20] demonstrated no improvement in regional perfusion as measured using a thermal imaging camera following TMR with a holmium:YAG laser in the distribution of an acutely ligated diagonal coronary artery in sheep. Malekan *et al.* [21]

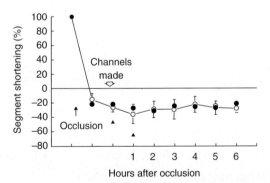

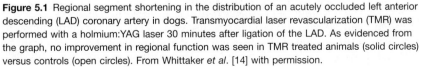

Figure 5.1 Regional segment shortening in the distribution of an acutely occluded left anterior descending (LAD) coronary artery in dogs. Transmyocardial laser revascularization (TMR) was performed with a holmium:YAG laser 30 minutes after ligation of the LAD. As evidenced from the graph, no improvement in regional function was seen in TMR treated animals (solid circles) versus controls (open circles). From Whittaker *et al.* [14] with permission.

ligated the LAD and second diagonal coronary arteries of sheep; in the experimental group, TMR was performed with a CO_2 laser immediately prior to coronary ligation. No difference in regional function was seen in control versus TMR treated sheep up to 8 weeks postoperatively.

Porcine models

Swine models have increasingly become the animal of choice for studies investigating not only TMR but other modes of therapeutic angiogenesis [22]. One advantage of swine is that their coronary anatomy, with minimal pre-existing coronary collateral vessels, is similar to that of humans [23]. One of the earliest studies of the effects of TMR on acutely ischemic myocardium was performed by Goda *et al.* [24], who used a low-power CO_2 laser to create channels in the anterior wall of the left ventricle of pigs immediately following ligation of multiple branches of the LAD coronary artery. Mortality was higher in TMR treated animals versus controls and there was no difference in the degree of left ventricular dysfunction between groups 3 weeks postoperatively. Mueller *et al.* [25] used a holmium:YAG laser to create TMR channels in the lateral wall of swine followed by ligation of several circumflex marginal arteries 30 minutes later. TMR failed to improve regional left ventricular function in the distribution of the circumflex coronary branches compared with controls at either 30 minutes or 1 month post-coronary occlusion. Similarly, Lutter *et al.* [26] performed CO_2 laser TMR prior to occlusion of the LAD in pigs and found no difference in regional perfusion to the LAD territory or left ventricular function 6 hours post-occlusion compared with untreated controls.

Summary

No study directly measuring regional myocardial blood flow after TMR performed in the setting of acute myocardial ischemia has found evidence for an immediate improvement in perfusion [13–16,19,20,26]. The findings of these studies in various acute cardiac ischemia models have provided clear evidence that TMR channels do not acutely improve regional myocardial blood flow, a tenet that is now widely accepted [1–3]. However, when the acute ischemic challenge was performed several months after creation of the TMR channels [7,8], a reduction in infarct size was observed, suggesting a delayed protective effect of TMR. These findings are consistent with a pro-angiogenic mechanism of action [2,3]. Similarly, greater long-term recovery of regional function in the territory of an occluded artery has been observed in TMR treated versus control animals in several studies [17,18], also suggestive of a delayed benefit, possibly as a result of angiogenesis.

Chronic ischemia models

Patients selected to undergo TMR generally have refractory angina pectoris and so-called "end-stage" coronary artery disease (CAD) [2]. This term refers to patients with the persistence of severe anginal symptoms (Canadian Cardiovascular Society class III and IV) despite maximal conventional antianginal combination therapy and coronary atherosclerosis not amenable to revascular-ization by percutaneous means or surgical bypass. The overwhelming majority of these patients has multivessel coronary disease and has undergone prior revascularization procedures [2]. These patients have ischemic yet viable my-ocardium as demonstrated by positron emission tomography (PET), thallium or technetium-sestamibi scintigraphy, magnetic resonance imaging (MRI), or dobutamine echocardiography. Patients eligible for TMR are frequently consid-ered to have areas of hibernating myocardium [2], although in reality many will have some combination of the various recognized clinical ischemic syndromes such as effort ischemia, chronic myocardial stunning, and chronic hibernation [22]. Consequently, chronic ischemia animal models are more appropriate for evaluating the effects of TMR on myocardial perfusion and function.

Rat models

Although rat models of chronic ischemia exist [5,27], few studies investigating the effects of TMR on myocardial perfusion and function have been performed using these models. Nahrendorf *et al.* [28] performed holmium:YAG TMR in re-mote myocardium 8 weeks after ligation of the left coronary artery in rats. Al-though not the area directly involved with infarct, hypertrophy of the remote region after MI in rats occurs in association with a reduction in capillary density in this remote area as well as reduced perfusion of the surviving myocardium [28]. Thus, this represents a model of chronic ischemia. Using this model, the in-vestigators found improved rest and stress perfusion, as measured using cine MRI, in the TMR treated remote areas compared with untreated controls. In addition, improved systolic wall thickening at rest as well as ejection fraction during dobutamine stress were seen in the TMR group. However, increased left ventricular dilatation and hypertrophy were seen in the TMR animals as well, suggestive of greater adverse left ventricular remodeling post-MI, changes the investigators potentially attributed to the large size of the laser channels relative to the small rat heart. The authors also suggested that MRI may be better suited to detection of small changes in perfusion after TMR, compared with the more widely utilized radionuclide techniques [28].

Canine models

As canine models of chronic ischemia have generally fallen out of favor in the past decade, little work has been carried out investigating TMR in chronic dog models. Yamamoto *et al.* [29] performed TMR with a holmium:YAG laser in the anterior wall of the left ventricle of dogs. During this same operation, they placed an ameroid constrictor on the LAD coronary artery and ligated all visible epicardial LAD collaterals. When the ameroid constrictor is implanted around an artery, the device absorbs water and swells compressing the artery and pro-ducing total coronary occlusion over a period of 14–30 or more days [22]. Be-cause of the gradual nature of the coronary occlusion with this device, collateral recruitment generally occurs such that regional myocardial blood flow at rest is preserved although coronary flow reserve is impaired such that ischemia results during periods of myocardial stress [22]. Consistent with this known property of the ameroid model, the study by Yamamoto *et al.* found no difference in regional myocardial blood flow at rest between the control and TMR treated animals as measured with colored microspheres 2 months post-ameroid placement. However, during adenosine-induced stress there was a significant increase in regional myocardial blood flow in the LAD distribution of the TMR treated animals (Fig. 5.2). Regional myocardial function was not assessed. This study was the first to demonstrate improved perfusion after TMR in a large animal model of chronic ischemia.

Ovine models

In the only chronic ovine study published to date, Ozaki *et al.* [30] used silastic snares to create 75% stenoses of the LAD and left circumflex (LCx) coronary arteries of sheep. Ten weeks later, animals randomized to TMR underwent creation of channels using a holmium:YAG laser on the anterior and posterior walls of the left ventricle. Twenty weeks after stenosis creation (10 weeks post-TMR in the experimental group), there was a significant increase in resting regional myocardial blood flow, as measured using colored microspheres, of the lased anterior and posterior walls of the left ventricle whereas no change was seen in

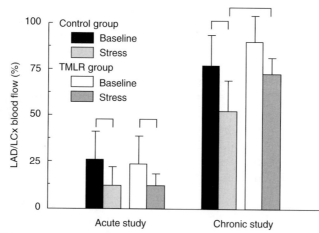

Figure 5.2 Regional myocardial blood flow in the distribution of the occluded left anterior descending (LAD) coronary artery expressed as a percentage of flow in the non-ischemic left circumflex (LCx) region. Immediately after temporary, acute occlusion of the LAD (labeled Acute Study in figure), there was no difference in regional myocardial blood flow at rest or during adenosine stress between TMR treated and untreated control dogs. These findings are consistent with the results of other acute ischemia studies outlined earlier in this chapter. Two months following gradual occlusion of the LAD by the ameroid constrictor (labeled Chronic Study in figure), there was a comparable increase in myocardial perfusion at rest in both control and TMR groups, consistent with the known property of collateral recruitment with the ameroid model. However, during adenosine stress, blood flow was significantly better maintained in the TMR group. Bars indicate pairs statistically different from each other ($P < 0.05$). From Yamamoto *et al.* [29] with permission.

untreated controls. Despite this increased blood flow, no improvement in either regional or global function was seen in the TMR animals versus controls up to 10 weeks post-TMR.

Porcine models

Porcine models of chronic ischemia have overwhelmingly become the most utilized for preclinical studies investigating therapeutic angiogenesis [22]. The most widely used porcine model of chronic ischemia has been the ameroid constrictor. These constrictors, when implanted around a coronary artery, absorb water and swell, producing total coronary occlusion over a period of several weeks [22].

Several studies investigating the effects of TMR on regional myocardial function and perfusion have been performed using the porcine ameroid model. Horvath *et al.* [31] placed ameroid constrictors around the LCx coronary artery of swine. Six weeks later, baseline rest and stress epicardial echocardiography was performed followed by TMR. Regional function was then re-assessed an additional 6 weeks after TMR. TMR treated LCx myocardium demonstrated a significant improvement in regional contractility at rest compared with untreated controls. However, no improvement in regional function during dobutamine stress was seen. Myocardial blood flow was not measured in this study. In a follow-up study [32], this same group compared laser TMR with an excimer laser with mechanical TMR using either a hot (50°C) needle, a normothermic needle, or an ultrasonic needle to create transmyocardial channels. Six weeks post-treatment, a significant improvement in regional function measured using epicardial echocardiography was observed in the laser TMR group only (Fig. 5.3). Martin *et al.* [33] compared the effects of CO_2 and excimer laser TMR on regional

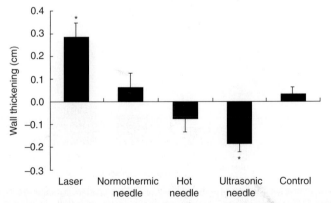

Figure 5.3 Regional myocardial wall thickening by epicardial echocardiography 6 weeks after treatment of left circumflex (LCx) myocardium with various transmyocardial revascularization devices or no device (control) in swine with LCx ameroid constrictors in place. Data are presented as change in wall thickening from pretreatment to 6 weeks post-treatment. Note significant improvement in regional function only in laser treated group. * $P < 0.01$ pretreatment vs post-Rx. After Horvath *et al.* [32] with permission.

myocardial perfusion and function in swine following proximal LCx ameroid constrictor placement. Three months after TMR, similar significant increases in regional myocardial perfusion, as measured using radioactive microspheres, were seen in both the CO_2 and excimer groups compared with untreated controls. Likewise, regional function, assessed using sonomicrometric techniques, was improved in both groups of TMR animals versus controls. Using the same porcine LCx ameroid constrictor model, Hamawy *et al.* [34] demonstrated a dose–response relationship between channel density and regional perfusion 4 weeks after TMR with an excimer laser. Animals receiving 50 channels in the LCx distribution had a significant improvement in myocardial blood flow during stress as measured using ^{99m}Tc-sestamibi perfusion scanning, whereas no significant improvement was seen with either 10 or 25 channels in the LCx region (Fig. 5.4).

Because of limitations of the ameroid constrictor model as a mimic of human coronary disease [35], including generally normal resting perfusion and function in the distribution of the occluded artery resulting from collateral recruitment, other models have been employed. Mühling *et al.* [36] used another coronary occlusion model involving placement of a hollow bead into the proximal LCx of swine via cardiac catheterization. The bead then gradually occludes the vessel over a period of 10 days post-implantation, not unlike the ameroid constrictor. One week after bead implantation, baseline MRI was performed to assess regional rest and stress perfusion and function. Animals were then randomized to TMR with a CO_2 laser or no treatment. Eight weeks following bead implantation (7 weeks post-TMR), the MRI studies were repeated. In untreated controls, there was a significant reduction in regional rest and stress perfusion

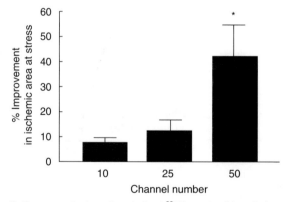

Figure 5.4 Quantitative computer-based analysis of ^{99m}Tc-sestamibi perfusion scans obtained 4 weeks after TMR compared with corresponding value immediately before lasing (3 weeks post-ameroid placement). Data are presented as percent improvement in adenosine stress-induced ischemia. A significant improvement was seen in only those animals receiving 50 channel TMR suggesting a dose–response relationship related to channel number may be important in TMR therapy. * $P = 0.05$. From Hamawy *et al.* [34] with permission.

1–8 weeks following bead implantation, corresponding to the occurrence of LCx occlusion during this time period. However, in the TMR treated animals, both rest and stress perfusion were preserved compared with the untreated group. Rest perfusion in the TMR animals was not significantly different from normal non-ischemic animals, although perfusion reserve was significantly reduced. Regional function in the LCx distribution improved significantly in the TMR treated animals and was not significantly different from normal non-instrumented animals, whereas no change was seen in untreated controls. Likewise, stroke volume and cardiac output were significantly reduced without TMR, but preserved in the TMR treated group. Finally, percent infarct assessed using triphenyltetrazolium chloride (TTC) staining was significantly less in the TMR treated versus untreated animals.

In our laboratory, we have developed a model of chronically ischemic yet viable (hibernating) myocardium involving placement of an adjustable occluder around the proximal LCx coronary artery to produce a high-grade stenosis of the artery. This model differs from the aforementioned chronic porcine models in that the artery remains patent with preserved antegrade flow through the LCx [37,38]. Consequently, collateral recruitment appears to be less than with total occlusion models [22]. Using PET to measure regional myocardial blood flow and dobutamine stress echocardiography to assess function, a significant increase in regional perfusion (Fig. 5.5a) was seen in areas treated with holmium:YAG or CO_2 laser 6 months post-TMR [39]. This increased perfusion was paralleled by a trend towards improved rest function and a significant improvement in regional wall motion during peak dobutamine stress (Fig. 5.5b). No improvement in either perfusion or function was seen in the control group 6 months after redo thoracotomy. A subsequent study using this model compared regional perfusion and function 6 months after TMR with holmium:YAG, CO_2, and xenon-chloride excimer lasers [40]. Improved blood flow was seen in the holmium:YAG and CO_2 treated animals 6 months post-TMR, whereas no significant change was seen after excimer TMR. As in the prior study, there was a trend towards improved rest function and a significant improvement in regional stress function in the holmium:YAG and CO_2 treated animals with no change in the excimer group. Finally, in a study comparing holmium:YAG laser TMR with mechanical transmyocardial revascularization using a transmyocardial implant device, improved LCx regional perfusion and function were seen only in the laser group 6 months post-treatment [41].

Conclusions

Chronic myocardial ischemia models in rats, dogs, sheep, and pigs have all demonstrated improved myocardial perfusion weeks to months after TMR using various techniques including radioactive [33] and colored [29,30] microspheres, ^{99m}Tc-sestamibi perfusion scanning [34], MRI [28], and PET [39–41] to directly measure regional myocardial blood flow. These experimental data

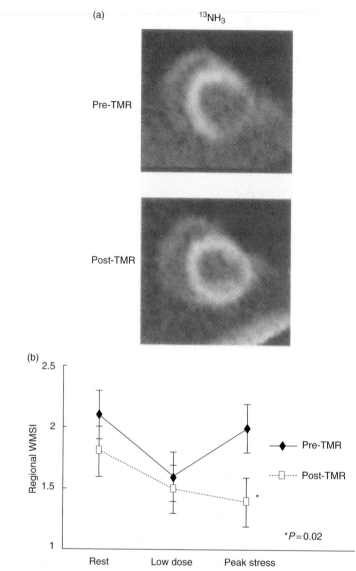

Figure 5.5 (a) Regional perfusion measured by ^{13}N-ammonia positron emission tomography (PET). Top image demonstrates reduced flow in distribution of stenotic left circumflex (LCx) coronary artery. Corresponding 6 month post-TMR scan from the same animal in bottom image demonstrates increased ^{13}N-ammonia accumulation consistent with improved blood flow. (b) Regional wall motion score index (WMSI) (1 = normal, with higher numbers indicating worsening function) at rest, low, and peak dobutamine stress for the LCx distribution before and 6 months after TMR. Note trend toward improved resting function and the significant improvement in regional WMSI at peak stress 6 months after TMR. From Hughes *et al.* [39] with permission.

provide clear evidence that TMR increases regional perfusion long-term in the treated regions. In addition, these studies have generally demonstrated some degree of improvement in either rest or stress function in association with the increased perfusion.

However, these results beg the question as to why clinical trials of TMR have not consistently demonstrated improvements in perfusion in the TMR treated patients. One potential explanation holds that the conventional nuclear imaging techniques (i.e., thallium, sestamibi) used in those clinical trials not demonstrating improved perfusion after TMR have lower spatial resolution and assess perfusion only semiquantitatively, thus limiting their ability to detect small changes in myocardial perfusion in patients with end-stage CAD [28,36]. Improvements in perfusion in human subjects may be too small to be detected with radionuclide scanning yet still be able to decrease the pain of angina pectoris [28,36]. Thus, some have suggested that MRI with its significantly higher spatial resolution and potential for quantification of myocardial perfusion may be better suited to detection of perfusion changes within and around the regions of TMR channel remnants [28,36]. MRI has been useful in experimental studies in detecting improved myocardial blood flow after TMR [28,36]. Preliminary clinical data suggest that MRI may also be superior to nuclear perfusion scans. Laham *et al.* [42] utilized MRI to examine 15 patients undergoing percutaneous holmium:YAG TMR and found a significant improvement in regional perfusion in the lased areas at 30 days and 6 months post-treatment despite no change in nuclear perfusion scans in these same patients.

Another potential explanation for the discrepancy between the human clinical and experimental animal studies involves differences in the potential of humans and animals to respond to TMR with new blood vessel growth in the treated regions. As alluded to above and discussed in further detail elsewhere in this book, many authors now feel that some form of angiogenesis represents the mechanism of action of TMR [2,3]. Consequently, human subjects with so-called "end-stage" CAD may lack the appropriate angiogenic substrate to respond to TMR in a manner analogous to experimental animals [22]. As outlined in this chapter, the experimental models typically utilized in preclinical studies of TMR involve young, healthy animals with single vessel coronary disease where the remaining vessels are normal and thus potentially more able to sprout collateral vessels capable of improving myocardial blood flow to the ischemic regions. These differences may explain the disparate results seen to date in animal versus human studies.

Finally, the chronic ischemia experimental studies have suggested that the technique employed in channel creation may be important. At least two studies [32,41] examining mechanical versus laser therapy for TMR in chronic ischemic models have demonstrated laser to be superior with regards to improvements in regional perfusion and function. This likely relates to the amount of injury and inflammation produced with each technique as well as possibly unknown thermoacoustic factors specific to laser therapy, which may lead to greater angiogenic growth factor upregulation. This is supported by the findings of a dose–response effect with an excimer laser in a porcine ameroid constrictor model [34]. Differences between lasers have also been demonstrated [40] and further work is needed to determine optimal laser operating parameters for the goal of therapeutic angiogenesis and explore means to improve on the current results of TMR.

References

1 Huikeshoven M, Beek JF, van der Sloot JAP, *et al.* 35 years of experimental research in transmyocardial revascularization: what have we learned? *Ann Thorac Surg* 2002;**74**:956–70.

2 Hughes GC, Abdel-aleem S, Biswas SS, Landolfo KP, Lowe JE. Transmyocardial laser revascularization: experimental and clinical results. *Can J Cardiol* 1999;**15**:797–806.

3 Hughes GC, Lowe JE. Revascularization versus denervation: what are the mechanisms of symptom relief? In: Abela GS, (ed.) *Myocardial Revascularization: Novel Percutaneous Approaches*. New York: Wiley-Liss, 2002: 63–79.

4 Hearse DJ. The elusive coypu: the importance of collateral flow and the search for an alternative to the dog. *Cardiovasc Res* 2000;**45**:215–9.

5 Doggrell SA, Brown L. Rat models of hypertension, cardiac hypertrophy, and failure. *Cardiovasc Res* 1998;**39**:89–105.

6 Guo JX, Pan J, Ma L, *et al.* Experimental studies of laser myocardial revascularization in rats. *Chin Med J* 1993;**106**:665–7.

7 Whittaker P, Rakusan K, Kloner RA. Transmural channels can protect ischemic tissue: assessment of long-term myocardial response to laser- and needle-made channels. *Circulation* 1996;**93**:143–52.

8 Whittaker P, Spariosu K, Ho Z-Z. Success of transmyocardial laser revascularization is determined by the amount and organization of scar tissue produced in response to initial injury: results of ultraviolet laser treatment. *Lasers Surg Med* 1999;**24**:253–60.

9 Mirhoseini M, Cayton MM. Revascularization of the heart by laser. *J Microsurg* 1981;**2**:253–60.

10 Okada M, Shimizu K, Ikuta H, Horii H, Nakamura K. A new method of myocardial revascularization by laser. *Thorac Cardiovasc Surg* 1991;**39**:1–4.

11 Jeevanandam V, Auteria JS, Oz MC, *et al.* Myocardial revascularization by laser-induced channels. *Surg Forum* 1990;**41**:225–7.

12 Yano OJ, Bielefeld MR, Jeevanandam V, *et al.* Prevention of acute regional ischemia with endocardial laser channels. *Ann Thorac Surg* 1993;**56**:46–53.

13 Landreneau R, Nawarawong W, Laughlin H, *et al.* Direct CO_2 laser "revascularization" of the myocardium. *Lasers Surg Med* 1991;**11**:35–42.

14 Whittaker P, Kloner RA, Przyklenk K. Laser-mediated transmural myocardial channels do not salvage acutely ischemic myocardium. *J Am Coll Cardiol* 1993;**22**:302–9.

15 Kohmoto T, Fisher PE, Gu A, *et al.* Does blood flow through holmium:YAG transmyocardial laser channels ? *Ann Thorac Surg* 1996;**61**:861–8.

16 Kohmoto T, Fisher PE, Gu A, *et al.* Physiology, histology, and 2-week morphology of acute transmyocardial channels made with a CO_2 laser. *Ann Thorac Surg* 1997;**63**:1275–83.

17 Kadipasaoglu KA, Pehlivanoglu S, Conger JL, *et al.* Long- and short-term effects of transmyocardial laser revascularization in acute myocardial ischemia. *Lasers Surg Med* 1997;**20**:6–14.

18 Horvath KA, Smith WJ, Laurence RG, *et al.* Recovery and viability of an acute myocardial infarct after transmyocardial laser revascularization. *J Am Coll Cardiol* 1995;**25**:258–63.

19 Eckstein FS, Scheule AM, Vogel U, *et al*. Transmyocardial laser revascularization in the acute ischaemic heart: no improvement of acute myocardial perfusion or prevention of myocardial infarction. *Eur J Cardiothorac Surg* 1999;**15**:702–8.

20 Eckstein FS, Scheule AM, Paunez Y, *et al*. Transmyocardial laser revascularization with the holmium:YAG laser does not improve myocardial perfusion in the acutely ischemic heart: an experimental study measuring myocardial perfusion by a thermal imaging camera. *Thorac Cardiovasc Surg* 1999;**47**:293–7.

21 Malekan R, Kelley ST, Suzuki Y, *et al*. Transmyocardial laser revascularization fails to prevent left ventricular functional deterioration and aneurysm formation after acute myocardial infarction in sheep. *J Thorac Cardiovasc Surg* 1998;**116**:752–62.

22 Hughes GC, Post MJ, Simons M, Annex BH. Porcine models of human coronary artery disease: implications for pre-clinical trials of therapeutic angiogenesis. *J Appl Physiol* 2003;**94**:1689–701.

23 Maxwell MP, Hearse DJ, Yellon DM. Species variation in the coronary collateral circulation during regional myocardial ischemia: a critical determinant of the rate of evolution and extent of myocardial infarction. *Cardiovasc Res* 1987;**21**:737–46.

24 Goda T, Wierzbicki Z, Gaston A, *et al*. Myocardial revascularization by CO_2 laser. *Eur Surg Res* 1987;**19**:113–7.

25 Mueller XM, Tevaearai HH, Genton C-Y, Bettex D, von Segesser LK. Transmyocardial laser revascularization in acutely ischaemic myocardium. *Eur J Cardiothorac Surg* 1998;**13**:170–5.

26 Lutter G, Yoshitake M, Takahashi N, *et al*. Transmyocardial laser-revascularization: experimental studies on prolonged acute regional ischemia. *Eur J Cardiothorac Surg* 1998;**13**:694–701.

27 Verdouw PD, van den Doel MA, de Zeeuw S, Duncker DJ. Animal models in the study of myocardial ischaemia and ischaemic syndromes. *Cardiovasc Res* 1998;**39**:121–35.

28 Nahrendorf M, Hiller K-H, Theisen D, *et al*. Effect of transmyocardial laser revascularization on myocardial perfusion and left ventricular remodeling after myocardial infarction in rats. *Radiology* 2002;**225**:487–93.

29 Yamamoto N, Kohmoto T, Gu A, *et al*. Angiogenesis is enhanced in ischemic canine myocardium by transmyocardial laser revascularization. *J Am Coll Cardiol* 1998;**31**:1426–33.

30 Ozaki S, Meyns B, Racz R, *et al*. Effect of transmyocardial laser revascularization on chronic ischemic hearts in sheep. *Eur J Cardiothorac Surg* 2000;**18**:404–10.

31 Horvath KA, Greene R, Belkind N, *et al*. Left ventricular functional improvement after transmyocardial laser revascularization. *Ann Thorac Surg* 1998;**66**:721–5.

32 Horvath KA, Belkind N, Wu I, *et al*. Functional comparison of transmyocardial revascularization by mechanical and laser means. *Ann Thorac Surg* 2001;**72**:1997–2002.

33 Martin JS, Sayeed-Shah U, Byrne JG, *et al*. Excimer versus carbon dioxide transmyocardial laser revascularization: effects on regional left ventricular function and perfusion. *Ann Thorac Surg* 2000;**69**:1811–6.

34 Hamawy AH, Lee LY, Samy SA, *et al*. Transmyocardial laser revascularization dose response: enhanced perfusion in a porcine ischemia model as a function of channel density. *Ann Thorac Surg* 2001;**72**:817–22.

35 Domkowski PW, Hughes GC, Lowe JE. Ameroid constrictor versus hydraulic occluder: creation of hibernating myocardium. *Ann Thorac Surg* 2000;**69**:1984.

36 Mühling OM, Wang Y, Panse P, *et al*. Transmyocardial laser revascularization preserves regional myocardial perfusion: an MRI first pass perfusion study. *Cardiovasc Res* 2003;**57**:63–70.

37 Hughes GC, Landolfo CK, Yin B, *et al*. Is chronically dysfunctional yet viable myocardium distal to a severe coronary stenosis hypoperfused? *Ann Thorac Surg* 2001;**72**:163–8.

38 St.Louis JD, Hughes GC, Kypson AP, *et al*. An experimental model of chronic myocardial hibernation. *Ann Thorac Surg* 2000;**69**:1351–7.

39 Hughes GC, Kypson AP, St.Louis JD, *et al*. Improved perfusion and contractile reserve after transmyocardial laser revascularization in a model of hibernating myocardium. *Ann Thorac Surg* 1999;**67**:1714–20.

40 Hughes GC, Kypson AP, Annex BH, *et al*. Induction of angiogenesis after TMR: a comparison of holmium:YAG, CO_2, and excimer lasers. *Ann Thorac Surg* 2000;**70**:504–9.

41 Hughes GC, Biswas SS, Yin B, *et al*. A comparison of mechanical and laser transmyocardial revascularization for induction of angiogenesis and arteriogenesis in chronically ischemic myocardium. *J Am Coll Cardiol* 2002;**39**:1220–8.

42 Laham RJ, Simons M, Pearlman JD, Ho KKL, Baim DS. Magnetic resonance imaging demonstrates improved regional systolic wall motion and thickening and myocardial perfusion of myocardial territories treated by laser myocardial revascularization. *J Am Coll Cardiol* 2002;**39**:1–8.

CHAPTER 6

Selection criteria for sole therapy and adjunctive therapy in combination with coronary artery bypass graft surgery

Charles R Bridges and Kapil Gopal

Introduction

Because of the progressive increase in the acuity of patients referred for coronary artery bypass surgery and the explosion in the number of percutaneous interventions (PCI) performed for coronary artery disease, an increasing percentage of patients with chronic, severe angina that persists despite maximal medical therapy can no longer be completely revascularized using either PCI or coronary artery bypass graft surgery (CABG). Most of these patients will have already undergone PCI or CABG and most will have relatively diffuse coronary artery disease. As a result, typically, the coronary anatomy precludes complete revascularization by either CABG or PCI. In other cases, complete revascularization may be achieved with CABG, but the risk : benefit ratio of CABG is prohibitive; for example, patients with patent internal mammary artery grafts who have only one graftable territory and intractable angina. If these patients have significant other comorbid conditions such as renal failure or chronic pulmonary disease, CABG may not be an attractive option. Transmyocardial revascularization (TMR) as sole therapy may be appropriate for some of these patients, and in others, it may be appropriate to perform TMR in combination with CABG or PCI. In this chapter we outline the currently accepted indications for TMR. We hope to provide a practical clinical guide with specific recommendations for the selection of patients for surgical TMR.

We will use the classification system format established in previous American College of Cardiology/American Heart Association and Society of Thoracic Surgeons Guidelines for diagnostic and therapeutic procedures:

1 *Class I:* Conditions for which there is evidence and/or general agreement that a given procedure or treatment is useful and effective

2 *Class II:* Conditions for which there is conflicting evidence and/or a divergence of opinion about the usefulness/efficacy of a procedure or treatment

- *IIA:* weight of evidence/opinion is in favor of usefulness/efficacy
- *IIB:* usefulness/efficacy is less well established by evidence or opinion

3 *Class III:* Conditions for which there is evidence and/or general agreement that the procedure/treatment is not useful and in some cases may be harmful

The level of evidence was assigned using the following criteria:
- A: Data derived from multiple randomized clinical trials
- B: Data derived from a single randomized trial or from several non-randomized studies
- C: Consensus expert opinion

The recommendations in this chapter are closely modeled after the clinical guidelines for TMR published by the Society of Thoracic Surgeons (STS) [1].

Background

The nature of the connections between the lumina of the ventricles and the coronary arteries is discussed extensively in several of the other chapters in this book. Vieussens in 1706 described "fleshy vessels" thought to represent direct communications between left ventricular myocardium and the left cardiac chambers [2] and, in 1708, Thebesius described connections between the interior of the cardiac chambers and the coronary venous network [3]. The existence of the thebesian veins is well accepted, but the debate about the existence and significance of direct "arterio-luminal" communications rages on [4,5]. There clearly is an unequivocal anatomic precedent for these connections, both in primitive vertebrate hearts, such as the single-chambered hearts of hagfish and lampreys, and reptilian hearts that are partially supplied by blood from the ventricular cavity [6,7]. Perhaps more relevant to TMR, it is well know in the pediatric cardiac surgical arena that patients with pulmonary atresia, intact ventricular septum, and proximal obstruction of the coronary arteries often have lumen-dependent myocardial perfusion [8]. Wearn's classic description of myocardial microanatomy [4] stimulated Vineberg, Pifarre, Sen, and others to develop new techniques for directly delivering oxygenated blood to the myocardium [9–15].

Lasers used for TMR

Mirhoseini *et al.* used a 450-W industrial carbon dioxide laser more than two decades ago to create transmyocardial channels in a canine model of acute ischemia and he was also the first to use the technique clinically as an adjunct to CABG and to demonstrate the safety of the technique [16,17]. The CO_2 laser available for clinical use required multiple pulses of energy to be delivered to create a transmural channel. As a result, at least one complete cardiac cycle was necessary to create a transmyocardial channel and the heart was required to be motionless during channel creation. This limitation made it necessary to perform the procedure under conditions of ischemic arrest [17].

TMR was initially thought to exert its effects via a direct supply of oxygenated blood to the myocardium from the left ventricular lumen. However, most experimental and autopsy series show that in fact the channels are closed shortly after creation [18–30]. Thus, the indications for TMR are based on its clinical efficacy in spite of the fact that its mechanism of action has not been clearly defined. There is an increasing quantity of experimental data that indicate, however, that angiogenesis may be one important mechanism underlying the clinical benefits of TMR [23,31,32] and although mechanical injury of the myocardium also induces an angiogenic response [21], laser TMR appears to provide an even greater stimulus for new blood vessel growth [32].

In 1990, engineers at PLC Systems, Franklin, MA, completed development of an 800–1000 W CO_2 laser. This laser, in contrast to the CO_2 laser employed by Mirhoseini, was specifically designed with sufficient pulse energy to allow for creation of transmyocardial channels in the left ventricle in approximately 40 ms, a period of time that is small compared with the normal cardiac cycle, allowing for successful creation of a transmural channel while the heart is still beating. The important engineering accomplishment of Robert Redko and others at PLC led to the first clinical trial of TMR. Other investigators utilized solid state lasers for experimental TMR, including the thulium-holmium-chromium:yttrium-aluminium-garnet (THC:YAG) laser and the holmium:YAG laser [33,34]. Most recently, the excimer laser has been utilized in clinical trials [35,36].

Both the CO_2 laser (PLC Systems, Franklin, MA) and the holmium:YAG laser (Cardiogenesis, Foothill Ranch, CA) are Food and Drug Administration (FDA) approved for clinical use. Light of the wavelength emitted by the CO_2 laser (10.6 µm) is more efficiently absorbed by water molecules than the light emitted by the holmium:YAG laser (wavelength 2.1 µm). The CO_2 laser allows the user to select the energy per pulse (20–80 J), and only one pulse is necessary to create a transmural channel. With the holmium:YAG laser, multiple pulses are required to generate a transmural channel, requiring delivery during several cardiac cycles. This approach also requires a small amount of mechanical energy as the fiber is manually advanced through the myocardium.

Clinical applications of TMR

Angina relief

Clinical studies of TMR using ether a CO_2 laser or the holmium:YAG laser have consistently demonstrated a marked reduction in angina symptoms and an improvement in exercise tolerance and quality of life [37–54]. The consistency of the clinical benefit of TMR as sole therapy in terms of angina reduction is overwhelming. Furthermore, these data include a number of randomized trials with follow-up extending to more than 5 years with consistent and sustained angina relief [46–54].

TMR when used as an adjunct to CABG has been more difficult to evaluate because CABG alone results in excellent angina relief and therefore confounds the assessment of the benefits of TMR in this setting. In an analysis of results obtained from the STS National Cardiac Database (NCD) for procedures performed between January 1998 and December 2001, Peterson *et al.* [55] reported the results of 2475 patients who underwent TMR (holmium:YAG and CO_2 laser combined) with concomitant CABG with a perioperative mortality of 4.2%. These authors also compared CABG/TMR patients with triple vessel disease but only one or two bypass grafts with similar patients in the STS NCD who underwent CABG alone, and found no significant difference in risk-adjusted mortality. This study has been criticized, however, because the "control" group may not have had the same incidence of diffuse coronary artery disease as the TMR/CABG group [56]. Stamou *et al.* [57] reviewed the results of CO_2 laser TMR plus CABG in 169 patients at the Washington Hospital Center. There were significant improvements in angina class during the follow-up period. After 12 months, only 4% of the patients were in Canadian Cardiovascular Society (CCS) class III or IV versus 90% of the patients preoperatively ($P < 0.001$) [57]. However, the operative mortality rate of 8.4% was not significantly different than the predicted mortality based on the STS NCD multivariable model for CABG alone (8.9%).

Allen *et al.* [58] reported the results of a prospective, randomized, multicenter trial of holmium:YAG TMR combined with CABG versus CABG alone for 263 patients with ungraftable myocardial segments. In this study, the ungraftable areas were treated with TMR in the TMR plus CABG arm and were left ungrafted in the CABG alone arm. These authors reported a significant reduction in the perioperative mortality rate (1.5% versus 7.6%) in the patients treated with TMR. At 1 year, the survival for patients in the TMR plus CABG group was 95% but only 89% in the CABG only group ($P = 0.05$). More recently, at 5-year follow-up, there was no mortality benefit for patients treated with TMR plus CABG compared with those treated with CABG alone, but there was a sustained, significant but small improvement in angina relief in patients who were treated with adjunctive TMR [56].

Procedural morbidity and mortality

Mortality
In the largest retrospective analysis of TMR results, 661 patients underwent TMR alone (holmium:YAG and CO_2 laser combined) with a perioperative mortality of 6.4%. For patients who underwent TMR with concomitant CABG, the mortality was 4.2%. In the prospective, randomized trials of CO_2 laser TMR, procedural mortality ranged from 3% to 5% with 1-year survival of 85–89% [38,46,47,50–52]. In the two prospective, randomized trials of holmium:YAG TMR, the procedural mortality ranged from 1% to 5% with 1-year survival of 89–96% [48,49].

In each of the randomized studies, patients with ejection fractions less than 20–30% were excluded, possibly accounting for the lower perioperative mortality rate observed when compared with several retrospective studies. In the study by Peterson *et al.* [55], mortality was significantly higher in patients with unstable angina or myocardial infarction (MI) within 21 days. Furthermore, in the 661 patients in the TMR-only group, the 143 patients without unstable angina and with ejection fractions >50% had an operative mortality of only 2.1%. Thus, patient selection is an important factor influencing acute mortality after TMR.

Morbidity

Morbidity from TMR may include myocardial infarction, arrhythmias, papillary muscle damage, left ventricular dysfunction, and cerebral microembolization. In experimental studies, holmium:YAG laser TMR resulted in an acute decrease in left ventricular systolic function [59] and with sufficient channel density, CO_2 laser TMR also may result in an acute decrease in left ventricular function [60]. Both types of laser TMR may result in significant increases in myocardial water content and impaired diastolic relaxation [59]. In the study by Peterson et al. [55], using data derived from the STS NCD for patients who underwent TMR as sole therapy, the incidence of major morbidity included reoperation for any reason (2.7%); stroke (0.76%); renal failure (4.8%); and prolonged ventilation (7.7%). In randomized trials of TMR as sole therapy, the incidence of CHF was 12–32%; MI, 7–18%, and arrhythmias occurred in 8–22% [38,46–52]. In an analysis of 49 patients who underwent CO_2 laser TMR enrolled in the Norwegian randomized trial, Tjomsland et al. [61] found a transient but significant decrease in cardiac index that was maximal immediately after the procedure. Four patients (8%) had an MI, seven patients (14%) developed atrial fibrillation, and two patients (4%) had ventricular arrhythmias. In a study of 21 patients who underwent CO_2 laser TMR by Hughes et al. [62], all patients had elevations in CPK and CPK-MB levels, and 54% of patients had ischemic changes on electrocardiogram in the first 48 hours after TMR.

Risk factors for morbidity and mortality following TMR

Unstable angina

In the randomized trial by Frazier et al. [50], more than 70% of the patients who crossed over to TMR from the medical treatment arm had unstable angina, and these patients had the highest perioperative mortality rate (9%). In the study by Hughes et al. [63], the presence of unstable angina was also a significant predictor of postoperative morbidity and mortality. In a multicenter study by Hattler et al. [64], perioperative mortality was 16% in patients with unstable angina compared with 3% in patients with chronic angina, and in the study based on data from the STS NCD, unstable angina was a significant risk factor for operative mortality [55].

Global myocardial ischemia

Burkhoff et al. [65] investigated the effects of age, sex, ejection fraction, prior CABG, unstable angina, and an index described as the anatomic myocardial perfusion index (AMP) as possible predictors of mortality after CO_2 laser TMR as sole therapy in 132 patients. They graded each vascular territory as AMP = 1 if there was unobstructed blood flow through a major artery to that territory and AMP = 0 if there was not. Patients with at least one territory with AMP = 1 had a mortality of 5% while those with AMP = 0 in all territories had a mortality of 25% (*P* = 0.002) [65]. Only AMP was a significant risk factor for operative mortality in the multivariate analysis. Kraatz *et al.* [66] found that mortality was highest in patients who underwent TMR alone or TMR plus CABG in whom, after the procedure, there was neither a patent bypass graft nor a native coronary artery perfusing at least one of the three major perfusion zones.

Diminished left ventricular function

Higher mortality after TMR has also been observed in patients with impaired left ventricular function or hemodynamic instability and limited reserve [67]. The use of a preoperative intra-aortic balloon pump in patients with unstable angina or reduced ejection fraction may be a useful adjunct to laser TMR [67].

It is important to note that patients with unstable angina, acute ischemia, and low ejection fraction have the highest risk of perioperative complications from sole therapy TMR. However, when TMR is combined with CABG, the literature provides little information regarding specific risks and benefits of adjunctive TMR.

Recommendations for TMR as sole therapy

Class I

TMR is indicated in patients with an ejection fraction greater than 30% and CCS class III or IV angina that is refractory to maximal medical therapy. These patients should have reversible ischemia of the left ventricular free wall and coronary artery disease corresponding to the region of myocardial ischemia. In all regions of the myocardium, the coronary disease must not be amenable to CABG or PCI, due to: (a) severe diffuse disease; (b) lack of suitable targets for complete revascularization; or (c) lack of suitable conduits for complete revascularization. (*Level of Evidence: A*)

Class IIB

The benefit of TMR is less well established in patients who otherwise have class I indications for TMR but who have either:
(a) Ejection fraction less than 30% with or without insertion of an intra-aortic balloon pump. (*Level of Evidence: C*)
(b) Unstable angina or acute ischemia necessitating intravenous antianginal therapy. (*Level of Evidence: B*)
(c) Patients with class II angina. (*Level of Evidence: C*)

Class III

TMR is not indicated in the following situations:
1 Patients without angina or with class I angina. (*Level of Evidence: C*)

2 Acute evolving myocardial infarction or recent transmural or non-transmural myocardial infarction. (*Level of Evidence: C*)

3 Cardiogenic shock defined as a systolic blood pressure less than 80 mmHg or a cardiac index of less than 1.8 L/min/m². (*Level of Evidence: C*)

4 Uncontrolled ventricular or supraventricular tachyarrythmias. (*Level of Evidence: C*)

5 Decompensated congestive heart failure. (*Level of Evidence: C*)

Recommendations for TMR as an adjunct to CABG

Class IIA
Adjunctive TMR is reasonable in:
Patients *with angina* (class I–IV) in whom CABG is the standard of care who also have at least one accessible and viable ischemic region with demonstrable coronary artery disease that cannot be bypassed, either due to: (a) severe diffuse disease; (b) lack of suitable targets for complete revascularization; or (c) lack of suitable conduits for complete revascularization. (*Level of Evidence: B*)

Class IIB
The usefullness of adjunctive TMR is less well established in:
Patients *without angina* in whom CABG is the standard of care who also have at least one accessible and viable ischemic region with demonstrable coronary artery disease which cannot be bypassed, either due to: (a) severe diffuse disease; (b) lack of suitable targets for complete revascularization; or (c) lack of suitable conduits for complete revascularization. (*Level of Evidence: C*)

Class III
Adjunctive TMR is not indicated in:
Patients in whom CABG is not the standard of care. (*Level of Evidence: C*)

References

1 Bridges CR, Allen KB, Horvath KA, *et al*. The Society of Thoracic Surgeons Practice Guideline Series/Transmyocardial laser revascularization: a report from the Society of Thoracic Surgeons Workforce on Evidence-Based Surgery. *Ann Thorac Surg* 2004;**77**:1494–502.

2 Vieussens R. *Nouvelles Découvertes Sur le Coeur*. Paris, 1706.

3 Thebesius AC. Disputatio medica de circulo sanguinis in corde. *Lugduni Batavorum*. 1708.

4 Wearn JT, Mettier SR, Klump TG, Zschiesche AB. The nature of the vascular communications between the coronary arteries and the chambers of the heart. *Am Heart J* 1933;**9**:143–70.

5 Tsang JC-C, Chiu RC-J. The phantom of "myocardial sinusoids": a historical reappraisal. *Ann Thorac Surg* 1995;**60**:1831–5.

6 Jensen D. The hagfish. *Sci Am* 1966;**214**:82–90.

7 Webb GJW. Comparative anatomy of the reptilia. III. The heart of crocodilians and a hypothesis on the completion of the interventricular septum of crocodilians and birds. *J Morphol* 1979;**161**:221–40.

8 Bonnet D, Gautier-Lhermitte I, Bonhoeffer P, Sidi D. Right ventricular myocardial sinusoidal–coronary artery connections in critical pulmonary valve stenosis. *Pediatr Cardiol* 1998;**19**:269–71.

9 Vineberg AM. Development of an anastamosis between the coronary vessels and a transplanted internal mammary artery. *Can Med Assoc J* 1946;**55**:117–9.

10 Pifarré R, Wilson SM, LaRossa DD, Hufnagel CA. Myocardial revascularization: arterial and venous implants. *J Thorac Cardiovasc Surg* 1968;**55**:309–19.

11 Goldman A, Greenstone SM, Preuss FS, Strauss SH, Chang ES. Experimental methods for producing a collateral circulation of the heart directly from the left ventricle. *J Thorac Surg* 1956;**31**:364–74.

12 Sen PK, Daulatram J, Kinare SG, Udwadia TE, Parulkar GB. Further studies in multiple transmyocardial acupuncture as a method of myocardial revascularization. *Surgery* 1968;**64**:861–70.

13 White M, Hershey JE. Multiple transmyocardial puncture revascularization in refractory ventricular fibrillation due to myocardial ischemia. *Ann Thorac Surg* 1968;**6**:557–63.

14 Pifarré R, Jasuja ML, Lynch RD, Neville WE. Myocardial revascularization by transmyocardial acupuncture: a physiologic impossibility. *J Thorac Cardiovasc Surg* 1969;**58**:424–31.

15 Massimo C, Boffi L. Myocardial revascularization by a new method of carrying blood directly from the left ventricular cavity into the coronary circulation. *J Thorac Surg* 1957;**34**: 257–64.

16 Mirhoseini M, Cayton MM: Revascularization of the heart by laser. *J Microsurg* 1981;**2**: 253–60.

17 Mirhoseini M, Shelgikar S, Cayton MM. New concepts in revascularization of the myocardium. *Ann Thorac Surg* 1988;**45**:415–20.

18 Burkhoff D, Fisher PE, Apfelbaum M, *et al*. Histologic appearance of transmyocardial laser channels after 4 1/2 weeks. *Ann Thorac Surg* 1996;**61**:1532–4.

19 Krabatsch T, Schaper F, Leder C, *et al*. Histological findings after transmyocardial laser revascularization. *J Cardiol Surg* 1996;**11**:326–31.

20 Gassler N, Wintzer HO, Stubbe HM, Wullbrand A, Helmchen U. Transmyocardial laser revascularization. Histological features in human nonresponder myocardium. *Circulation* 1997;**95**:371–5.

21 Malekan R, Reynolds C, Kelley ST, Suzuki Y, Bridges CR. Angiogenesis in transmyocardial laser revascularization: a non-specific response to injury. *Circulation* 1998;**98**(Suppl 2):62–5.

22 Malekan R, Kelley ST, Suzuki Y, *et al*. Transmyocardial laser revascularization fails to prevent left ventricular functional deterioration and aneurysm formation after acute myocardial infarction in sheep. *J Thorac Cardiovasc Surg* 1998;**116**:752–62.

23 Chu V, Giaid A, Kuang J, *et al*. Angiogenic response to transmyocardial revascularization (TMR): laser versus mechanical punctures. *Ann Thorac Surg* 1999;**68**:301–7; discussion 307–8.

24 Kohmoto T, Fisher P, Gu A, *et al*. Physiology, histology, and 2-week morphology of acute transmyocardial channels made with a CO_2 laser. *Ann Thorac Surg* 1997;**63**:1275–83.

25 Kohmoto T, Fisher P, Gu A, *et al*. Does blood flow through holmium:YAG transmyocardial channels? *Ann Thorac Surg* 1996;**61**:861–8.

26 Kohmoto T, DeRosa CM, Yamamoto N, *et al*. Evidence of vascular growth associated with laser treatment of normal canine myocardium. *Ann Thorac Surg* 1998;**65**:1360–7.

27 Fisher PE, Kohmoto T, DeRosa CM, *et al*. Histologic analysis of transmyocardial channels: comparison and CO_2 and holmium:YAG lasers: *Ann Thorac Surg* 1997;**65**:466–72.

28 Yamamoto N, Kohmoto T, Gu A, *et al*. Angiogenesis is enhanced in ischemic canine myocardium by transmyocardial laser revascularization. *J Am Coll Cardiol* 1998;**31**:1426–33.

29 Fleischer KJ, Goldschmidt-Clermont PJ, Fonger JD, *et al*. One-month histologic response of transmyocardial laser channels with molecular intervention. *Ann Thorac Surg* 1996;**62**: 1051–8.

30 Zlotnick AY, Ahmad RM, Reul RM, *et al*. Neovascularization occurs at the site of closed laser channels after transmyocardial laser revascularization. *Surg Forum* 1996;**XLVII**:286–87.

31 Horvath KA, Chiu E, Maun DC, *et al*. Upregulation of VEGF mRNA and angiogenesis after transmyocardial laser revascularization. *Ann Thorac Surg* 1999;**68**:825–9.

32 Horvath KA, Belkind N, Wu J, *et al*. Functional comparison of transmyocardial revascularization by mechanical and laser means. *Ann Thorac Surg* 2001;**72**:1997–2002.

33 Jeevanandam V, Auteri JS, Oz MC, *et al*. Myocardial revascularization by laser induced channels. *Surg Forum* 1990;**41**:225–7.

34 Yano OJ, Bielefeld MR, Jeevanandam V, *et al*. Prevention of acute regional ischemia with endocardial laser channels. *Ann Thorac Surg* 1993;**56**:46–53.

35 Lee LY, O'Hara MF, Finnin EB, *et al*. Transmyocardial laser revascularization with excimer laser: clinical results at 1 year. *Ann Thorac Surg* 2000;**70**:498–503.

36 van der Sloot JAP, Huikeshoven M, Tukkie R, *et al*. Transmyocardial revascularization using an XeCl excimer laser: results of a randomized trial. *Ann Thorac Surg* 2004;**78**:875–81.

37 Horvath KA, Cohn LH, Cooley DA, *et al*. Transmyocardial laser revascularization: results of a multicenter trial with transmyocardial laser revascularization used as sole therapy for end-stage coronary artery disease. *J Thorac Cardiovasc Surg* 1997;**113**:645–53.

38 Schofield, PM, Sharples LD, Caine N, *et al*. Transmyocardial laser revascularization in patients with refractory angina: a randomised controlled trial. *Lancet* 1999;**353**:519–24.

39 Cooley DA, Frazier OH, Kadipasaoglu KA, *et al*. Transmyocardial laser revascularization: clinical experience with twelve-month follow-up. *J Thorac Cardiovasc Surg* 1996;**111**:791–9.

40 Donovan CL, Landolfo KP, Lowe JE, *et al*. Improvement in inducible ischemia during dobutamine stress echocardiography after transmyocardial laser revascularization patients with refractory angina pectoris. *J Am Coll Cardiol* 1997;**30**:607–12.

41 Frazier OH, Cooley DA, Kadipasaoglu KA, *et al*. Myocardial revascularization with laser: preliminary findings. *Circulation* 1995;**92**(Suppl 2):58–65.

42 Horvath KA, Mannting F, Cummings N, Sherman SK, Cohn LH. Transmyocardial laser revascularization: operative techniques and clinical results at two years. *J Thorac Cardiovasc Surg* 1996;**111**:1047–53.

43 Krabatsch T, Tambeur L, Lieback E, Shaper F, Hetzer R. Transmyocardial laser revascularization in the treatment of end-stage coronary artery disease. *Ann Thorac Cardiovasc Surg* 1998;**4**:64–71.

44 Lutter G, Sauerbier B, Nitzsche E, *et al*. Transmyocardial laser revascularization (TMLR) in patients with unstable angina and low ejection fraction. *Euro J Cardiothoracic Surg* 1998;**13**:21–6.

45 Milano A, Pratali S, Tartarini G, *et al*. Early results of transmyocardial revascularization with a holmium laser. *Ann Thorac Surg* 1998;**65**:700–4.

46 Aaberge L, Nordstrand K, Dragsund M, *et al*. Transmyocardial revascularization with CO_2 laser in patients with refractory angina pectoris. Clinical results from the Norwegian randomized trial. *J Am Coll Cardiol* 2000;**35**:1170–7.

47 Aaberge L, Rootwelt K, Blomhoff S, *et al*. Continued symptomatic improvement three to five years after transmyocardial revascularization with CO_2 laser: a late clinical follow-up of the Norwegian randomized trial with transmyocardial revascularization. *J Am Coll Cardiol* 2002;**39**:1588–93.

48 Allen KB, Dowling RD, Fudge TL, *et al*. Comparison of transmyocardial revascularization with medical therapy in patients with refractory angina. *N Engl J Med* 1999;**341**:1029–36.

49 Burkhoff D, Schmidt S, Schulman SP, *et al.* Transmyocardial laser revascularization compared with continued medical therapy for treatment of refractory angina pectoris: a prospective randomized trial. *Lancet* 1999;**354**:885–90.

50 Frazier OH, March RJ, Horvath KA. Transmyocardial revascularization with a carbon dioxide laser in patients with end-stage coronary artery disease. *N Engl J Med* 1999;**341**:1021–8.

51 Horvath KA, Aranki SF, Cohn LH, *et al.* Sustained angina relief 5 years after transmyocardial laser revascularization with CO_2 Laser. *Circulation* 2001;**104**:181–4.

52 Horvath KA, Cohn LC, Cooley DA, *et al.* Transmyocardial laser revascularization: results of multi-center trial using TLR as sole therapy for end stage coronary artery disease. *J Thorac Cardiovasc Surg* 1997;**113**:645–54.

53 De Carlo M, Milano AD, Pratali S, *et al.* Symptomatic improvement after transmyocardial laser revascularization: how long does it last? *Ann Thorac Surg* 2000;**70**:1130–3.

54 Allen KB, Dowling RD, Angell WW, *et al.* Transmyocardial revascularization: 5-year follow up of a prospective, randomized multicenter trial. *Ann Thorac Surg* 2004;**77**:1228–34.

55 Peterson ED, Kaul P, Kaczmarek RG, *et al.* From controlled trials to clinical practice: monitoring transmyocardial revascularization use and outcomes. *J Am Coll Cardiol* 2003;**42**: 1611–6.

56 Allen KB, Dowling RD, Schuch DR, *et al.* Adjunctive transssmyocardial revascularization: five-year follow-up of a prospective, randomized trial. *Ann Thorac Surg* 2004;**78**:458–65.

57 Stamou SC, Boyce SW, Cooke RH, *et al.* One-year outcome after combined coronary artery bypass grafting and transmyocardial laser revascularization for refractory angina pectoris. *Am J Cardiol* 2002;**89**:1365–8.

58 Allen KB, Dowling RD, DelRossi AJ, *et al.* Transmyocardial laser revascularization combined with coronary artery bypass grafting: a multicenter, blinded, prospective, randomized, controlled trial. *J Thorac Cardiovasc Surg* 2000;**119**:540–9.

59 Hughes GC, Shah AS, Yin B, *et al.* Early postoperative change in regional systolic and diastolic left ventricular function after transmyocardial laser revascularization: a comparison of holmium:YAG and CO_2 lasers. *J Am Coll Cardiol* 2000;**35**:1022–30.

60 Mouli SK, Fronza J, Greene R, Robert ES, Horvath KA. What is optimal channel density for transmyocardial laser revascularization. *Ann Thorac Surg* 2004;**78**:1326–31.

61 Tjomsland O, Aaberge L, Almdahl S, *et al.* Perioperative cardiac function and predictors for adverse events after transmyocardial laser treatment. *Ann Thorac Surg* 2000;**69**:1098–103.

62 Hughes GC, Landolfo KP, Lowe JE, Coleman RB, Donovan CL. Diagnosis, incidence, and clinical significance of early postoperative ischemia after transmyocardial laser revascularization. *Am Heart J* 1999;**137**:1163–8.

63 Hughes GC, Landolfo KP, Lowe JE, Coleman RB, Donovan CL. Perioperative morbidity and mortality after transmyocardial laser revascularization: incidence and risk factors for adverse events. *J Am Coll Cardiol* 1999;**33**:1021–6.

64 Hattler BG, Griffith BP, Zenati MA, *et al.* Transmyocardial laser revascularization in the patient with unmanageable unstable angina. *Ann Thorac Surg* 1999;**68**:1203–9.

65 Burkhoff D, Wesley MN, Resar JR, Lansing AM. Factors correlating with risk of mortality after transmyocardial revascularization. *J Am Coll Cardiol* 1999;**34**:55–61.

66 Kraatz EG, Misfeld M, Jungbluth B, Sievers HH. Survival after transmyocardial laser revascularization in relation to nonlasered perfused myocardial zones. *Ann Thorac Surg* 2001;**71**:53206.

67 Lutter G, Saurbier B, Nitzsche E, *et al.* Transmyocardial laser revascularization (TMLR) in patients with unstable angina and low ejection fraction. *Eur J Cardiothorac Surg* 1998; **13**:21–6.

CHAPTER 7

Results of prospective randomized trials

Keith B Allen and Keith A Horvath

Introduction

A majority of patients with angina related to coronary artery disease (CAD) respond to medical management (MM), percutaneous coronary intervention (PCI), or coronary artery bypass grafting (CABG). However, there is a growing number of patients who have medically refractory angina caused by diffuse CAD who are not eligible for conventional revascularization [1] or who would be incompletely revascularized by CABG alone [2]. Transmyocardial revascularization (TMR) has yielded positive clinical results in these difficult subsets of patients.

Reports from five prospective, randomized clinical trials, designed to evaluate the safety and effectiveness of TMR as sole therapy for the treatment of medically refractory, stable angina have appeared in the literature [3–7]. The positive results [3,4] led to the US Food and Drug Administration approval of a holmium:yttrium-aluminum-garnet (Ho:YAG) laser system (CardioGenesis Corporation, Foothill Ranch, CA) and a carbon dioxide (CO_2) laser system (PLC Medical Systems, Franklin, MA). More recently, 3–5 year follow-up of these trials is becoming available [8–10]. In addition to using TMR in the treatment of stable angina, its use in the management of unstable angina has been reported [3,4,11–14]. Furthermore, each laser system has been evaluated in a multicenter, prospective, randomized trial for TMR as an adjunct to CABG in patients who would be incompletely revascularized by CABG alone [15,16]. This chapter reviews the clinical science surrounding TMR with an emphasis on the randomized controlled trials performed in these patient groups.

TMR laser systems

Ho:YAG system
The CardioGenesis Ho:YAG laser system is a pulsed laser with a maximum energy output of 20 W. Laser calibrations deliver 6–8 W per laser pulse at a rate of five pulses per second through a 1-mm diameter flexible fiberoptic bundle. When TMR is used as sole therapy, anesthesia includes a short-acting inhalation agent supplemented with low-dose narcotics and propofol. Intravenous fluids

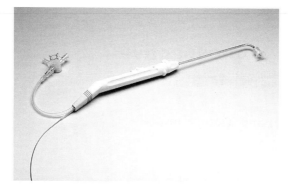

Figure 7.1 The CardioGenesis SoloGrip®III TMR Handpiece.

are minimized to avoid fluid overloading. The distal two-thirds of the left ventricle is exposed using a limited left anterolateral thoracotomy through the fifth intercostal space. The SoloGrip® III hand piece allows the surgeon to position and stabilize the embedded fiberoptic bundle (CrystalFlex® fiber) against the epicardial surface (Fig. 7.1). Energy delivery of 6–10 pulses is typically required to traverse the myocardium and is controlled with a foot switch. Laser channels are placed every square centimeter in the distal two-thirds of the left ventricle, avoiding obviously scarred areas. After the placement of 3–5 channels, digital pressure is applied for 1–2 minutes to obtain hemostasis and allow for myocardial recovery. Epicardial ligation of a laser channel for persistent bleeding is rarely required. Intraoperative arrhythmias are unusual if channels are placed slowly and mechanical manipulation of the heart is minimized. Laser energy, when absorbed by ventricular blood, produces an acoustic image analogous to steam that is readily visible by transesophageal echocardiography (TEE). Initially, TEE can be used to confirm penetration of the laser into the left ventricle. After several procedures, however, tactile and auditory feedback enables surgeons to confirm transmural penetration without TEE.

CO_2 system

The PLC CO_2 laser system (Fig. 7.2) has a maximum energy output of 1000 W and is set to deliver 800 W in pulses 1–99 ms long at energies of 8–80 J to create 1 mm diameter channels. Typical operative settings are 20 J per pulse of 25–40 ms duration. Energy is delivered via an operator-set articulated arm and handpiece placed against the epicardial surface. Transmural channels are created with a single pulse.

When the CO_2 system is used for sole therapy, patient positioning and surgical approach to the heart are similar to that described above. The CO_2 system uses helium-neon laser guidance for epicardial positioning of the handpiece, and electrocardiographic (ECG) synchronization to fire on the R-wave of the ECG cycle when the ventricle is maximally distended and electrically quiescent. TEE is used to confirm transmural penetration.

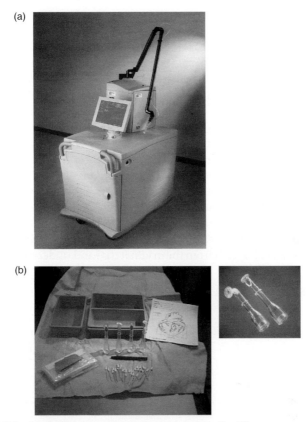

Figure 7.2 (a) The CO_2 Heart Laser. (b) CO_2 Laser Revascularization Kit.

TMR as an adjunct to CABG is performed with or without cardiopulmonary bypass (CPB). If CPB is used, it is preferred to perform adjunctive TMR with the Ho:YAG system on an arrested heart just after initiating CPB. This minimizes intraoperative arrhythmias and may reduce bleeding compared with placing laser channels at the conclusion of CPB [8]. CO_2 TMR in conjunction with CABG on CPB can be performed either before or after the grafts have been completed while the heart is beating. During off-pump CABG cases, TMR is typically performed after bypass grafts are completed.

Trial designs and results

TMR as sole therapy in stable patients

Trial designs
The safety and effectiveness of Ho:YAG and CO_2 TMR laser systems as sole therapy have been evaluated in five prospective, randomized, clinical trials (three

multicentered and two single-centered) for the treatment of patients with medically refractory stable angina whose anatomy was not amenable to CABG or PCI [3–7]. Experimental designs and patient selection criteria among the trials were similar. Study endpoints included operative (in-hospital or to 30 days) mortality and 1-year survival; improvement in angina class; myocardial perfusion; exercise tolerance; quality of life; cardiac-related hospitalization; and major adverse cardiac events. Aside from a variation in the number of patients, certain features made each trial unique (Table 7.1). Whereas Allen *et al.* [3] randomized patients with medically refractory class IV angina only, varying proportions of patients with class III and IV angina were enrolled in the remaining trials [4–7]. Two trial designs permitted cross-over from the MM to the TMR arm provided the *a priori* treatment failure criteria were met (hospitalized and unweanable from intravenous antianginal medications [IVAA] for 48 hours). Of the patients initially randomized to the MM arm in Allen *et al.* [3] and Frazier *et al.* [4], 32% (46/143) and 59% (60/101), respectively, met the treatment failure criteria and were withdrawn from the original trial and underwent TMR while

Table 7.1 Randomized controlled trials of sole therapy transmyocardial revascularization (TMR).

Characteristic*	Allen et al. [3]	Frazier et al. [4]	Burkhoff et al. [5]	Schofield et al. [6]	Aaberge et al. [7]
Trial design	TMR vs. MM, 1 : 1 randomization				
System used	Ho:YAG	CO_2	Ho:YAG	CO_2	CO_2
Number of centers	18	12	16	1	1
Patients (n)	275	192	182	188	100
Cross-over allowed	Yes	Yes	No	No	No
Age† (years)	60	61	63	60	61
Male gender (%)	74	81	89	88	92
EF†‡ (%)	47	50	50	48	49
Class III/IV§ (%)	0/100	31/69	37/63	73/27	66/34
CHF (%)	17	34	nr	9	nr
Diabetes (%)	46	40	36	19	22
Hyperlipidemia (%)	79	57	77	nr	76
Hypertension (%)	70	65	74	nr	28
Prior MI¶ (%)	64	82	70	73	70
Prior CABG (%)	86	92	90	95	80
Prior PCI (%)	48	47	53	29	38
No. of channels‡	39	36	18	30	48

CABG, corony artery bypass graft; EF, ejection fraction; Ho, holmium; MI, myocardial infarction; MM, medical management; nr, not reported; PCI, percutaneous coronary intervention; YAG, yttrium-aluminium-garnet.
* Demographic characteristics listed for patients randomized to TMR.
† Mean or median.
‡ Left ventricular ejection fraction.
§ Canadian Cardiovascular Society (CCS) class [3–6]; New York Heart Association (NYHA) class [7].
¶ Myocardial infarction.

unstable. In the remaining three trials [5–7], cross-over from the MM to the TMR arm was not allowed, thus simplifying statistical analyses and data interpretation.

Operative mortality and long-term survival

Operative mortality and 1-year survival rates observed in the five prospective, randomized trials are summarized in Table 7.2. Operative mortality following TMR in stable patients ranged from 1% to 5%. The low rate (1%) reported by Burkhoff *et al.* [5] was attributed to strict study enrollment criteria that excluded patients with no region of protected myocardium (defined as a vascular territory perfused by unobstructed – no lesion with >50% stenosis – blood flow through a major native vessel or bypass graft), left main stenosis >50%, or a change in angina symptoms or medication usage in the preceding 21 days. Allen *et al.* [3] reported a reduced operative mortality rate from 5% overall to 2% in the last 100 consecutively randomized patients, attributable to refinement of surgical technique involving judicious intraoperative fluid management, postoperative diuresis, allowance for myocardial recovery following the placement of 3–5 laser channels, and withholding of β-blockers and calcium-channel blockers for 48 hours post-TMR. Additional information regarding a predictor of perioperative mortality was gleaned from the trial by Frazier *et al.* [4]. In that study, patients who underwent TMR within 1 week of an episode of unstable angina requiring intravenous heparin and nitroglycerine had a 22% mortality rate. If the patients were stabilized, able to be weaned off the medications, and were treated with TMR 2 weeks later the perioperative mortality rate was 1%. This operative mortality rate is similar to that reported by the Society of Thoracic Surgeons (STS) for patients undergoing CABG alone (approximately 2%) [17].

Kaplan–Meier 1-year survival rates for randomized groups within each of the five trials were statistically similar. One-year survival ranged from 84% to 95% in TMR patients, and from 79% to 96% in medically managed patients. Longer

Table 7.2 Operative mortality and 1-year survival in randomized, controlled trials of sole therapy transmyocardial revascularization (TMR).

Studies	Number randomized		Operative mortality*	1-year Kaplan–Meier survival[†]	
	TMR	MM	TMR	TMR	MM
Allen *et al.* [3]	132	143	5%	84%	89%
Frazier *et al.* [4]	91	101	3%	85%	79%
Burkhoff *et al.* [5]	92	90	1%	95%	90%
Schofield *et al.* [6]	94	94	5%	89%	96%
Aaberge et al. [7]	50	50	4%	88%	92%

MM, medical management.
* Operative: days 0–30.
[†] No statistically significant differences between groups.

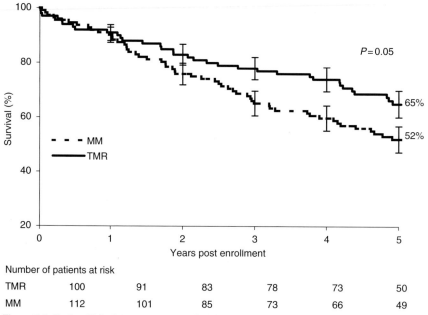

Figure 7.3 Kaplan–Meier intent-to-treat survival through 5 years following randomization to treatment with Ho:YAG transmyocardial revascularization (TMR) or medical management (MM).

term survival, which is a key component to establishing the risk : benefit profile of any innovative treatment, has been evaluated in randomized patients in two of these studies. Aaberge *et al.* [8], utilizing a CO_2 system, reported similar survival rates among 75 randomized patients with primarily class III angina at a mean of 43 months (78% vs. 76%, TMR vs. MM; P = ns). In a 5-year follow-up of 212 randomized patients, all with class IV angina, Allen *et al.* [9] reported increased Kaplan–Meier survival for patients randomized to Ho:YAG TMR versus MM (65% vs. 52%; P = 0.05; Fig. 7.3), with a significantly lower annualized mortality rate beyond 1 year (8% vs. 13%, TMR vs. MM; P = 0.03).

Effectiveness of therapy

Angina improvement at 1 year

Significant angina improvement (defined as a reduction of two or more angina classes from baseline) was observed through 1 year following TMR as compared with MM in each of the randomized trials (P <0.001) [3–7]. The percentage of TMR-treated patients with at least a two-class improvement in angina at 1 year varied from 25% to 76%, and is related to the proportion of patients enrolled in each study who had baseline class IV angina (Fig. 7.4). Allen *et al.* [3] and Frazier *et al.* [4], with the highest proportions of patients with baseline class IV angina (100% and 69%, respectively) reported at least two-class angina improvement in 76% and 72% of TMR patients, respectively. Schofield *et al.* [6], with the lowest proportion of baseline class IV patients (23%), reported angina improvement in

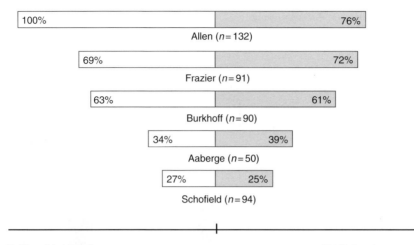

Figure 7.4 Angina improvement 1 year following transmyocardial revascularization (TMR) by proportion in class IV at baseline. *n*, Number of patients randomized to TMR.

only 25% of TMR patients which was still significantly better then the 4% improvement noted in the MM arm.

In each of the five randomized trials, maximal medical therapy was comparable between randomized groups at baseline, although it is recognized that there is not one defined regimen that is constant from patient to patient. In each of these trials, a significant reduction in antianginal medication usage at 12 months was observed in TMR patients versus MM controls [3–7]. The significant angina relief following TMR is not brought about by medication, but in fact results in a decrease in requisite antianginal drugs.

Long-term angina improvement
Reports of long-term follow-up of prospectively randomized patients are available [8,9]. At a mean of 5 years, Allen *et al.* [9] evaluated the effectiveness of TMR in 212 "no option" patients originally randomized to TMR (*n* = 100) or to MM (*n* = 112). To eliminate the potential for assessment bias in this long-term follow-up, blinded independent assessors performed angina assessments across centers. Significantly more TMR than MM patients continued to experience at least two-class angina improvement from baseline (88% vs. 44%; $P < 0.001$) or were free from angina symptoms altogether (33% vs. 11%; $P = 0.02$) at a mean of 5 years (Fig. 7.5). Importantly, the investigators found that freedom from angina and 1-year angina improvement were highly predictive of long-term freedom from angina and the survival benefit observed in randomized TMR patients, respectively. No differences between groups in antianginal medication usage were observed. Aaberge *et al.* [8], in a single-center follow-up of 75 randomized patients using a CO_2 system, found that angina symptoms were still significantly improved (24% vs. 3%, TMR vs. MM; $P = 0.001$) and unstable angina

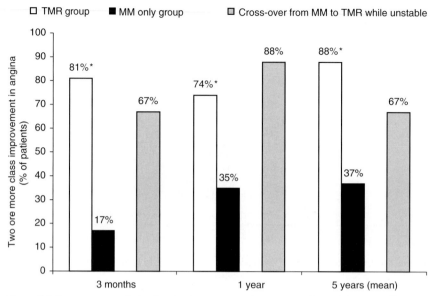

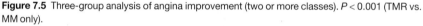

Figure 7.5 Three-group analysis of angina improvement (two or more classes). $P < 0.001$ (TMR vs. MM only).

hospitalizations were significantly reduced ($P < 0.05$) at a mean follow-up of 43 months. Additional long-term follow-up after CO_2 TMR reported by Horvath *et al.* [18] demonstrated sustained angina relief. After an average of 5 years and up to 7 years of follow-up, the average angina class was significantly improved from baseline and unchanged from 1 year postoperatively (Fig. 7.6). At 5 years, 81% of the patients were in class II or better and 17% had no angina. Using the two-class reduction in angina as a definition of success, 68% of the patients had successful long-term angina relief.

Exercise tolerance
Exercise tolerance time (ETT) was a primary endpoint in three trials [5–7]. Burk-hoff *et al.* [5] reported significantly improved median modified Bruce treadmill exercise tolerance times at 12 months (+65 vs. –46 seconds, TMR vs. MM; $P < 0.0001$). Moreover, at 1 year, a significant reduction in chest pain at peak exercise with no evidence of an increase in silent ischemia was observed when comparing TMR with MM patients [19]. Unique to this trial, investigators designed the ETT test to obtain evidence of angina refractory to medical treatment, to account for possible exercise habituation effects, and to ensure test reproducibility (minimum of two tests with durations varying by ≤15%) at baseline. The test could be limited by symptoms or ECG ischemic changes, but typical angina occurring during at least one test was required. In a single-center report, Schofield *et al.* [6] used a symptom-limited modified Bruce treadmill exercise test and a 12-minute walk test to characterize the effects of TMR versus continued MM on

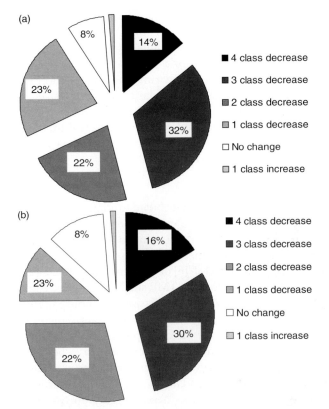

Figure 7.6 Angina class change: (a) from baseline to 5 years; (b) from baseline to 1 year.

exercise tolerance. At 1 year, mean adjusted treadmill time was 40 seconds longer in the TMR group than in the MM group ($P = 0.15$), and the test was stopped more frequently for angina among MM than TMR patients ($P < 0.001$). Mean 12-minute walk distance was 33 m further for TMR than MM patients ($P = 0.1$), and nitrate usage and frequency of angina during or after the walk were significantly lower in TMR than MM patients ($P \leq 0.04$). In another single-center report, Aaberge et al. [7] used an electrically braked cycle ergometer held at approximately 60 rpm for exercise testing. Time to onset of angina favored the TMR group, and angina was reported as an exercise-limiting factor in significantly fewer TMR patients.

Quality of life
Improved clinical status following TMR has been assessed in a variety of ways, including assessment of standardized quality of life measures, calculation of cardiac rehospitalization rates, or determination of event-free survival. Quality of life analyses using the Duke Activity Status Index [3] or the Seattle Angina Questionnaire [4,5] revealed that TMR patients enjoyed significantly improved quality of life at 1 year compared with MM patients. Similarly, significantly

reduced rates of cardiac-related rehospitalization through 1 year were reported for patients randomized to TMR versus MM [3,4,6]. Finally, consistent results have been reported for composite endpoints that strongly favor TMR over MM. Allen *et al.* [3] observed significantly increased cardiac event-free survival (defined as freedom from death, Q-wave myocardial infarction, cardiac-related rehospitalization, or subsequent revascularization attempt) at 1 year (54% vs. 31%, TMR vs. MM; $P < 0.001$). Using a different composite endpoint, Frazier *et al.* [4] observed significantly increased event-free survival (defined as freedom from death, Q-wave myocardial infarction, unstable angina, or class IV angina) at 1 year (66% vs. 11%, TMR vs. MM; $P < 0.001$).

Perfusion studies
The clinical benefit of TMR may be attributed to angiogenesis and improved or redistributed blood flow. Objective evidence of improved myocardial blood flow following TMR has been demonstrated. Employing technetium sestamibi:thallium scans to determine the areas of scar (fixed defects) and ischemia (reversible defects), Schofield *et al.* [6] demonstrated significant decrease in the number of reversible defects for both TMR and MM patients. The improvement in the ischemic areas in the TMR group was noted without a significant increase in the number of fixed defects over the year of follow-up. However, the number of fixed defects or infarcts in the MM group doubled over the same interval. Therefore TMR led to restoring normal perfusion in ischemic myocardium. Frazier *et al.* [4] reported a 20% improvement in the perfusion of previously ischemic areas in the TMR group and a 27% worsening of perfusion in ischemic areas of the MM group at 12 months. These changes were not caused by significant changes in the areas of scar for either group.

Placebo effect
Because none of the surgical trials comparing TMR with MM were blinded, it has been suggested that angina relief following TMR may have been the result of a placebo effect induced by the surgical incision. The scientific validation of a long-term placebo effect from a sham thoracotomy is limited [20]. The long-term, persistent benefits of surgical TMR observed by several studies [8–10] argue against a placebo effect. Whereas a placebo effect likely influences early outcomes in any clinical trial involving innovative technology, its persistence is diminished in late follow-up and is much less plausible in the long-term, especially in light of the observed survival benefit. The overwhelmingly positive 1-year results from four prospective randomized trials in which primarily class IV angina patients were enrolled [3–5,7], as well as the reported persistent significant angina relief beyond 3 years [8] and 5 years [9,10] following TMR mitigates the concern of placebo effect as a primary mechanism explaining the clinical benefits of TMR. Additionally, other objective data including the improvement in perfusion from the randomized trials as well as improvement in myocardial metabolism as documented by a positron emission tomography (PET) scan [21,22]. Functional improvement has also been demonstrated using dobuta-

mine stress echocardiography as well as CINE and contrast enhanced magnetic resonance imaging [23,24]. These demonstrations of functional improvement were accompanied by a decrease in myocardial ischemia without an increase in myocardial infarction in TMR treated patients. This evidence is not subject to the placebo effect.

Based on an assessment of the cumulative results from multiple randomized trials, the recently updated ACC/AHA guidelines [25] and recently developed STS guidelines [26] have determined that the weight of the evidence favors the use of TMR in the treatment of stable, medically refractory, no option angina patients.

TMR as sole therapy in unstable patients

In addition to using TMR for the treatment of patients with stable, medically refractory angina, several studies have evaluated it in a limited number of patients with unstable angina [3,4,11–14]. Enrollment criteria included diffuse CAD not amenable to CABG or PCI, inability to be weaned from IVAA after two or more attempts, and a left ventricular ejection fraction ≥25%. March *et al.* [11], Allen *et al.* [3,14], and Frazier *et al.* [4] reported results in patients who became unstable after being randomized to medical therapy as part of prospective trials. Hattler *et al.* [12] and Dowling *et al.* [13] reported on larger numbers of patients who initially presented with unstable angina and were treated with TMR.

Patients with unstable angina and without conventional interventional options represent a higher risk group for TMR. March *et al.* [11] and Hattler *et al.* [12], using the CO_2 laser system, and Dowling *et al.* [13] and Allen *et al.* [3], using the Ho:YAG laser system, reported operative mortality rates of 27%, 16%, 12%, and 9%, respectively, following TMR in unstable angina patients. Despite this finding, it has not been uncommon for cardiologists to delay referral of stable "no option" patients for TMR until they become unstable, often treating Canadian Cardiovascular Society (CCS) class IV patients with non-surgical alternatives such as enhanced external counterpulsation or investigational gene or drug therapies, which are perceived as less risky.

Hattler *et al.* and Allen *et al.* compared results following TMR in stable and unstable patients. Hattler *et al.* [12] compared the effect of sole therapy TMR in medically refractory patients with unstable angina ($n = 91$) and stable angina ($n = 76$). Operative mortality was higher in unstable versus stable patients (16% vs. 3%; $P = 0.005$); however, late mortality up to 1 year was similar (13% vs. 11%; $P = 0.83$). Angina improvement at 12 months was significantly improved in both groups from baseline ($P < 0.001$), and was comparable between groups, with approximately 50% of patients able to resume normal activity levels without angina. Allen *et al.* [3] compared TMR in 132 stable patients with 46 unstable "cross-over" patients (cross-over patients were initially randomized to medical therapy, met the *a priori* criteria for treatment failure, and crossed over to receive TMR while unstable). Operative mortality (5% vs. 9%; $P = 0.48$) and 1-year survival (84% vs. 91%; $P = 0.53$) were similar. At 5 years [9], whereas significant angina improvement persisted similarly in both TMR and cross-over patients, survival curves showed a diverging trend. In a three-group analysis, 5-year survival for patients randomized to TMR was 65%, compared with 53% and 48% ($P = 0.16$), respectively, for MM patients who did not cross-over and for those who did.

These long-term results raise a serious clinical question as to whether TMR treatment should be delayed once a no option patient with medically refractory, stable angina is identified. Allen *et al.* [9] found that histories of myocardial infarction and prior PCI were significant predictors of medical therapy treatment failure and subsequent cross-over; however, these were not predictive of mortality at 5 years. This suggests that in terms of long-term survival, randomization to the original TMR group is superior to crossing over to receive TMR after becoming unstable. While TMR has a defined operative risk, delaying TMR in identified stable candidates cannot be recommended because of the potential for increased operative mortality and reduced long-term survival.

TMR as an adjunct to CABG

Incomplete revascularization after CABG occurs in up to 25% of patients and represents a risk for late cardiac events [2,27–30]. In one series, the presence of diseased but non-grafted arteries posed a significant negative influence on event-free survival defined as the absence of death, recurrent angina, myocardial infarction, and the need for repeat CABG [28]. The safety and effectiveness of TMR combined with CABG have been difficult to assess because of the influence of bypass grafts and lack of randomized control arms in some studies [31,32].

To date, two prospective, randomized, multicentered trials have been performed using TMR adjunctively with CABG. In a single-blinded trial involving 263 patients, Allen *et al.* [15], using a Ho:YAG system, randomized patients whose standard of care was CABG but who had one or more viable myocardial target areas served by coronary vessels that were not amenable to bypass grafting to either CABG plus TMR (CABG/TMR; $n = 132$) or CABG alone ($n = 131$). Baseline and operative characteristics were similar between groups, with patients blinded to their treatment group through 1-year follow-up. The authors reported improved outcomes following CABG/TMR versus CABG alone in terms of a reduced operative mortality rate (1.5% vs. 7.6%; $P = 0.02$), reduced postoperative left ventricular support requirements, increased 30-day freedom from major adverse cardiac events (97% vs. 91%; $P = 0.04$), and improved 1-year Kaplan–Meier survival (95% vs. 89%; $P = 0.05$). Multivariable predictors of operative mortality were CABG alone (odds ratio [OR] 5.3; $P = 0.04$) and increased age (OR 1.1; $P = 0.03$). While the overall angina class distribution and exercise treadmill scores were similar between groups at 1 year, CABG/TMR patients tended to have less severe angina ($P = 0.2$). In a similar, smaller study using the CO_2 laser system, Frazier *et al.* [16] reported preliminary results from a prospective, multicentered trial that randomized 49 high-risk patients to CABG/TMR ($n = 22$) or CABG alone ($n = 28$). Compared with CABG alone, CABG/TMR tended to reduce operative mortality (9% vs. 33%; $P = 0.09$) and increase angina improvement at 1 year (63% vs. 34%; $P = 0.34$). As bypass grafts deteriorate, longer term follow-up will determine if adjunctive TMR slows the inevitable return of angina for patients not completely revascularized by CABG alone.

Early benefits observed in these studies following CABG/TMR must be evaluated in the context of potential study limitations. In both studies [15,16], randomization occurred preoperatively, potentially resulting in differences between groups in terms of characterization of bypassable vessels and surgical conduct. Allen *et al.* [15] reported similar operative characteristics between groups with respect to time on CPB, number and distribution of bypass grafts, and the rate of endarterectomy, suggesting groups were well matched. In addition, whereas the operative mortality rates observed following CABG alone in both studies (7.6%, 33%) might be viewed as excessive, the presence of diffuse CAD is currently not factored into commonly used models for predicting surgical risk; nonetheless, the evidence in the clinical literature indicates this is of vital importance. Graham *et al.* [30] concluded that diffuse CAD appropriately quantified is a powerful independent predictor of operative mortality. Furthermore, Osswald *et al.* [33] determined that incomplete revascularization in the elderly, because of small or diffusely diseased targets, is significantly predictive of operative mortality following CABG.

Additional retrospective data regarding the use of TMR as an adjunct to CABG further demonstrates the safety and efficacy of the procedure. Stamou *et al.* [24] reported the results of 169 TMR post-CABG patients performed at a single institution. Ninety percent of the patients were in class III or IV preoperatively and only 4% had significant angina 12 months postoperatively. The operative mortality rate was 8.4%, which was not significantly different to the predicted mortality based on the STS National Cardiac Database multivariable model for CABG alone (8.9%). Review of the STS National Cardiac Database from January 1998 to 2001, revealed that 2475 patients underwent TMR plus CABG. The perioperative mortality for those patients was 4.2%. The comparison from the database of patients who underwent CABG only who had three-vessel disease and less than three bypass grafts versus patients who had TMR plus CABG showed no significant difference in morbidity or mortality [34]. TMR plus CABG has been shown to decrease intensive care unit times and lengths of stay [35].

Conclusions

The results of multiple, randomized, controlled trials using Ho:YAG system and CO_2 TMR systems, and the recently available long-term follow-up data, validate the safety and effectiveness of TMR for the treatment of patients with severe angina resulting from diffuse CAD. The observed long-term persistence in angina improvement and survival benefits in identified stable patients support increased utilization of TMR. Adjunctive use of TMR with CABG is safe and may provide an additional method to provide a more complete revascularization for patients with severe coronary artery disease.

References

1 Muhkerjee D, Bhatt D, Roe T, Patel V, Ellis SG. Direct myocardial revascularization and angiogenesis: how many patients might be eligible? *Am J Cardiol* 1999;**84**:598–600.

2 Weintraub WS, Jones EL, Craver JM, Guyton RA. Frequency of repeat coronary bypass or coronary angioplasty after coronary artery bypass surgery using saphenous venous grafts. *Am J Cardiol* 1994;**73**:103–12.

3 Allen KB, Dowling RD, Fudge TL, *et al.* Comparison of transmyocardial revascularization with medical therapy in patients with refractory angina. *N Engl J Med* 1999;**341**:1029–36.

4 Frazier OH, March RJ, Horvath KA. Transmyocardial revascularization with a carbon dioxide laser in patients with end-stage coronary disease. *N Engl J Med* 1999;**341**:1021–8.

5 Burkhoff D, Schmidt S, Schulman SP, *et al.* Transmyocardial revascularization compared with continued medical therapy for treatment of refractory angina pectoris: a prospective randomized trial. *Lancet* 1999;**354**:885–90.

6 Schofield PM, Sharples LD, Caine N, *et al.* Transmyocardial laser revascularization in patients with refractory angina: a randomized controlled trial. *Lancet* 1999;**353**:519–24.

7 Aaberge L, Nordstrand K, Dragsund M, *et al.* Transmyocardial revascularization with CO_2 laser in patients with refractory angina pectoris. Clinical results from the Norwegian randomized trial. *J Am Coll Cardiol* 2000;**35**:1170–7.

8 Aaberge L, Rootwelt K, Blomhoff S, *et al.* Continued symptomatic improvement three to five years after transmyocardial revascularization with CO_2 laser: a late clinical follow-up of the Norwegian randomized trial with transmyocardial revascularization. *J Am Coll Cardiol* 2002;**39**:1588–93.

9 Allen KB, Dowling R, Angell W, *et al.* Transmyocardial revascularization: five-year follow-up of a prospective, randomized, multicenter clinical trial. *Ann Thorac Surg* 2004;**77**:1228–34.

10 Horvath KA, Aranki SF, Cohn LC, *et al.* Sustained angina relief 5 years after transmyocardial laser revascularization with a CO_2 laser. *Circulation* 2001;**I**:81–4.

11 March RJ, Boyce S, Cooley DA. Improved event free survival following transmyocardial laser revascularization versus medical management in patients with unreconstructed coronary artery disease. The 77th Annual Meeting of the American Association of Thoracic Surgery. 1997: 94 (abstract).

12 Hattler B, Griffith B, Zenati M, *et al.* Transmyocardial laser revascularization in the patient with unmanageable unstable angina. *Ann Thorac Surg* 1999;**68**:1203–9.

13 Dowling RD, Petracek MR, Selinger SL, Allen KB. Transmyocardial revascularization in patients with refractory, unstable angina. *Circulation* 1998;**98**(Suppl 2):73–6.

14 Allen KB, Dowling RD, Heimansohn DA, *et al.* Transmyocardial revascularization utilizing a holmium:YAG laser. *Eur J Cardiothorac Surg* 1998;**14**(Suppl 1):S100–4.

15 Allen KB, Dowling R, DelRossi A, *et al.* Transmyocardial laser revascularization combined with coronary artery bypass grafting: a multicenter, blinded, prospective, randomized, controlled trial. *J Thorac Cardiovasc Surg* 2000;**119**:540–9.

16 Frazier OH, Boyce SW, Griffith BP, *et al.* Transmyocardial revascularization using a synchronized CO_2 laser as adjunct to coronary artery bypass grafting: results of a prospective, randomized multi-center trial with 12 month follow-up. *Circulation* 1999;**100**(Suppl 1):248.

17 http://www.ctsnet.org/file/STSNationalDatabaseSpring2003ExecutiveSummary.pdf

18 Cooley DA, Frazier OH, Kadipasaoglu KA, *et al.* Transmyocardial laser revascularization: clinical experience with 12-month follow-up. *J Thorac Cardiovasc Surg* 1996;**111**:791–9.

19 Myers J, Oesterle S, Jones J, Burkhoff D. Do transmyocardial and percutaneous laser revascularization induce silent ischemia? An assessment by exercise testing. *Am Heart J* 2002;**143**:1052–7.

20 Allen KB, Shaar CJ. Transmyocardial laser revascularization as a clinical procedure. Letter to the editor. *N Engl J Med* 2000;**342**:438.

21 Kadipasaoglu KA, Frazier OH. Transmyocardial laser revascularization: effective laser parameters on tissue ablation and cardiac perfusion. *Semin Thorac Cardiovasc Surg* 1999; **11**:4–11.

22 Donovan CL, Landolfo KP, Lowe JE, *et al.* Improvement in inducible ischemia during dobutamine stress echocardiography after transmyocardial laser revascularization in patients with refractory angina pectoris. *J Am Coll Cardiol* 1997;**30**:607–12.

23 Horvath KA, Kim RJ, Judd RM, Parker MA, Fullerton DA. Contrast enhanced MRI assessment of microinfarction after transmyocardial laser revascularization. *Circulation* 2000; **102**(Suppl 2):765–8.

24 Stamou SC, Boyce SW, Cooke RH, *et al.* One-year outcome after combined coronary artery bypass grafting and transmyocardial laser revascularization for refractory angina pectoris. *J Am Coll Cardiol* 2002;**89**:1365–8.

25 Gibbons R, Abrams J, Chatterjee K, *et al.* ACC/AHA 2002 guideline update for the management of patients with chronic stable angina: summary article. A report of the American College of Cardiology/American Heart Association Task Force on Practice Guidelines (Committee on the Management of Patients with Chronic Stable Angina). *Circulation* 2003;**107**:149–58.

26 Bridges CR, Horvath KA, Nugent B, *et al.* Society of Thoracic Surgeons Workforce on Clinical Pathways: Transmyocardial Revascularization. *Ann Thorac Surg* 2004;**77**:1494–502.

27 Lawrie GM, Morris GC, Silvers A, *et al.* The influence of residual disease after coronary bypass on the 5-year survival rate of 1274 men with coronary artery disease. *Circulation* 1982;**66**:717–23.

28 Schaff H, Gersh B, Pluth J, *et al.* Survival and functional status after coronary artery bypass grafting: results 10 to 12 years after surgery in 500 patients. *Circulation* 1983;**68**(Suppl 2):200–4.

29 Bell, MR, Gersh BJ, Schaff HV, *et al.* Effect of completeness of revascularization on long-term outcomes of patients with three-vessel disease undergoing coronary artery bypass surgery. *Circulation* 1992;**86**:446–57.

30 Graham MM, Chambers RJ, Davies RF. Angiographic quantification of diffuse coronary artery disease: reliability and prognostic value for bypass operations. *J Thorac Cardiovasc Surg* 1999;**118**:618–27.

31 Trehan N, Mishra M, Bapna R, *et al.* Transmyocardial laser revascularization combined with coronary artery bypass grafting without cardiopulmonary bypass. *Eur J Cardiothorac Surg* 1997;**12**: 276–84.

32 Stanou S, Boyce S, Cooke R, *et al.* One-year outcome after combined coronary artery bypass grafting and transmyocardial laser revascularization for refractory angjna pectoris. *Am J Cardiol* 2002;**89**:1365–8.

33 Osswald B, Blackstone E, Tochtermann U, *et al.* Does the completeness of revascularization affect early survival after coronary artery bypass grafting in elderly patients? *Eur J Cardiothorac Surg* 2001;**20**:120–6.

34 Peterson ED, Kaul P, Kaczmarek RG, *et al.* Society of Thoracic Surgeons. From controlled trials to clinical practice: monitoring transmyocardial revascularization use and outcomes. *J Am Coll Cardiol* 2003;**42**:1611–6.

35 Wehberg KE, Julian JS, Todd JC, *et al.* Improved patient outcomes when transmyocardial revascularization is used as adjunctive revascularization. *Heart Surg Forum* 2003;**6**:329–30.

CHAPTER 8

Combination therapy with coronary artery bypass grafting

Kapil Gopal and Charles R Bridges

Introduction

Since the first use of transmyocardial laser revascularization (TMR) in the 1980s by Mirhoseini and Cayton in a canine model of acute ischemia, TMR has quickly become an approved method of revascularization in patients with refractory end-stage coronary artery disease (CAD). Originally thought to increase myocardial perfusion by direct blood flow through artificially created sinusoids connected to the left ventricular lumen, the actual mechanism of efficacy remains to be elucidated. Current hypotheses for the effects of TMR include stimulation of neo-angiogenesis and/or regional myocardial denervation.

Several randomized, controlled, multicenter trials have established the clinical efficacy of sole-therapy TMR [1–5]. The patients studied had advanced angina pectoris refractory to medical treatment with diffuse atherosclerotic lesions that were not amenable to percutaneous transluminal coronary angioplasty (PTCA) or coronary artery bypass grafting (CABG). In general, the trials demonstrated that treatment with TMR significantly increased exercise tolerance time, lowered Canadian Cardiovascular Society (CCS) angina scores, and improved patient perceptions of quality of life compared with continued maximal medical therapy alone after 1 year post-TMR follow-up. Recently published findings from 3–5 year follow-up of the same patients showed sustained angina relief that was superior and associated with significantly increased survival rates in the TMR group of patients compared with medical therapy alone [6–9].

Transmyocardial revascularization has become an increasingly popular mode of therapy. In a review, the Society of Thoracic Surgeons (STS) database reported an increase in STS institutions performing TMR from 33 (7% of total STS sites) in 1998 to 131 (36% of total STS sites) in 2001 [10]. There was a similar linear increase in the number of procedures performed during the same time frame, with a total of 3717 TMR procedures in the 3-year time period [10]. Of these, 2475 (67%) were combined CABG procedures with adjunctive use of TMR, whereas 661 (17%) were TMR-only procedures [10]. The remaining 581 procedures were TMR as an adjunct with some other cardiac procedure.

The clinical benefits associated with TMR as sole therapy were compelling enough to convince the Food and Drug Administration (FDA) to approve TMR as an acceptable method of revascularization in patients not suitable for traditional revascularization techniques, PTCA or CABG. However, the majority of reported incidence of TMR use was as an adjunct to CABG. Some studies of TMR in animal models of myocardial ischemia have demonstrated increased myocardial regional blood flow, reduction of infarct size, and preservation of contractile function compared with untreated controls [11].

Evidence

There have been several single-arm and comparative studies of TMR as an adjunct to CABG. Stamou *et al.* [13] reported on 169 patients receiving CABG plus TMR between 1996 and 2000 at a single institution. The group was followed at regular intervals for up to 12 months. Patients with intractable angina and ≥ 1 major vessel or branch surrounded by viable myocardium not amenable to surgical revascularization were included in the study. Anatomic targets too small or with severe diffuse atherosclerotic disease were deemed unsuitable for surgical revascularization. Patients with recent myocardial infarction, severe arrhythmias, and decompensated heart failure were excluded. The study illustrated sustained angina relief post-procedure as only 3% (5/169) of patients had CCS class III–IV angina after treatment at 3 months and only 4% (seven patients) at 6 and 12 months compared with 90% (152 patients) pretreatment. The use of cardioactive medication postoperatively declined from 91% pretreatment to 66% at 3 months, 54% at 6 months, and 56% at 12 months. At the end of the study, 81% were free of adverse cardiac events, an actuarial survival rate of 85% with an operative mortality of 8.2%. The study did not investigate mechanism of action.

Trehan *et al.* [14,15] found similarly encouraging results in two studies using TMR as an adjunct to CABG performed without the use of cardiopulmonary bypass. In both studies, TMR was performed in regions of ischemic viable myocardium with non-graftable vessels or to the lateral or inferior walls even when graftable targets were present. In one study, 56 patients underwent TMR plus CABG during a 14-month period with 50.99% of patients exhibiting CCS class III–IV angina preoperatively. The mean follow-up was 9.2 months with 90.9% patients remaining angina free at 12 months and mean exercise tolerance increased from 5.2 min pretreatment to 9.4 min at 12 months. In a follow-up study [15], 77 patients underwent TMR plus CABG over a 2-year period with similarly positive results. Mean follow-up for this group was 16.6 months, with 89% remaining angina free at 12 months and a similar increase in exercise tolerance as the earlier study. In the two studies, the TMR plus CABG groups exhibited 25% and 28% increases, respectively, in myocardial perfusion over 12 months as assessed by thallium-201 myocardial perfusion scintigraphy in the regions receiving TMR. Operative mortality was limited to only one patient in each series. Comparable results were seen in 17 patients who were considered to be high risk because of a previous CABG, a prior history of myocardial infarction, or advanced age (<70 years). In the high-risk group, mean follow-up was 6 months and one patient died prior to discharge [16].

Vincent et al. [17] concluded that TMR was a safe alternative method for revascularization in patients who were considered poor candidates for traditional bypass surgery. In this study, 268 patients with at least one ungraftable target region whom had typically been refused surgery at other centers were evaluated. Fifty-two percent of patients were deemed not to be candidates for conventional (CABG) revascularization and underwent TMR only. In 48% only incomplete revascularization was possible and these patients formed the TMR plus CABG group. Both groups included subjects who also underwent staged performance of PTCA, TMR via endoscopic or "minimally invasive" techniques, and TMR to the septum. However, no conclusions were derived from these specific variations in technique. The TMR-alone group received on average 33.15 channels and the TMR plus CABG group received on average 3.16 bypass grafts along with 22 channels per patient. Hospital mortality rate for TMR-alone patients was 9.3% (12/128 patients) and TMR plus CABG was 11.8% (15/127 patients). Postoperatively, 80.8% of all patients had CCS scores of 0–1. In contrast, 93% of patients had CCS scores of 3–4 prior to treatment. After the 12-month follow-up period, 82% of patients in the TMR plus CABG group had CCS scores of 0–1 compared with only 42% of the TMR-alone cohort. During the same period, 45% and 17% of the TMR-alone and combined groups, respectively, reverted to CCS scores of 3–4. Eighty-eight percent of the entire study population reported improved quality of life. Improved exercise tolerance was seen without improved cardiac function by cardiac scintigraphy. Echocardiographic evaluation of left ventricular contractile function showed improvement in 78% and 96% at 12 months in the TMR-alone and combined therapy groups, respectively. Based on these findings, Vincent et al. [17] concluded that TMR as sole therapy or adjunctive therapy is suitable when all other measures have been exhausted. Diegeler et al. [18] conducted a similar study with a smaller cohort of patients (28 patients in total: 16 patients in TMR-only group, and 12 patients in combined TMR and CABG group) using the holmium:YAG laser. Their findings were similar to Vincent et al. with dramatically lower angina scores, increased exercise tolerance, and acceptable mortality rate postoperatively in both groups. Myocardial scintigraphy and echocardiography did not demonstrate improved ejection fraction or myocardial perfusion in TMR-treated areas.

Wehberg et al. [19] compared the effectiveness of CABG alone with CABG plus TMR in 255 patients requiring revascularization for severe CAD. A total of 219 were completely revascularized by CABG and the remaining 36 had CABG plus TMR performed in regions with non-graftable targets. All patients had ≥30% ejection fraction and CCS class III–IV angina. After comparing 30-day outcomes for the two groups, Wehberg et al. concluded that in-hospital outcomes were improved in the TMR plus CABG group versus the CABG alone group. All patients had a similar number of grafts performed and operating room times, but the intensive care unit and total length of hospitalization times were significantly shorter in the CABG plus TMR group (2.1 ± 0.2 days versus 1.6 ± 0.2 days ($P < 0.001$) and 8.2 ± 0.4 days versus 7.1 ± 0.6 days, respectively). The frequency of postoperative atrial fibrillation was significantly lower (37.4% versus 16.7%;

$P < 0.025$) and the readmission rate was also lower (7.8% versus 2.8%) in the TMR- plus CABG group.

Three randomized controlled trials (RCTs) have been widely cited in studying the effectiveness of TMR as an adjunct to CABG versus CABG alone [20–22]. The first trial was published as an abstract only by Frazier *et al.* in 1999 [21]. A small group of patients ($n = 49$) were included from five surgical centers and were considered to be high-risk for perioperative mortality with CABG. There was a non-significant trend towards decreased perioperative mortality in the combined therapy group when compared with CABG-only patients. The trial by Loubani *et al.* [22] of CABG plus TMR versus CABG only studied the effects of each treatment strategy on angina class and exercise tolerance. The patients had no history of myocardial infarction, normal left ventricular function, and at least one non-graftable artery. The patients ($n = 20$) were randomly divided into two groups and followed up at 6, 18, and 36 months. Both groups had similar numbers of grafts and the time on cardiopulmonary bypass was comparable. There was no significant difference seen between the two groups in anginal class through the follow-up period. However, the greater improvement in exercise tolerance seen in the TMR plus CABG versus the CABG-alone group at 6 months (199.2 ± 66.5 s per patient versus 46.8 ± 20.0 s, respectively) was sustained at 18 months (157 ± 46.3 s versus 61 ± 39.2 s), but not at 36 months (57.2 ± 42.1 s versus 68.1 ± 46.7 s).

The largest RCT published by Allen *et al.* [20] enrolled 263 patients with isolated CAD and viable myocardial regions with one or more major vessels not suitable for bypass. The study was conducted at 24 centers and the patients were prospectively randomized and blinded for up to 12 months. Immediately postoperatively, the TMR plus CABG patients required less inotropic support (33% versus 55%). The most significant benefit seen was a significant reduction in operative mortality with the use of adjunctive TMR with CABG when compared with CABG alone (1.5% [2/131] versus 7.5% [10/132]). This benefit persisted until the completion of the study at 12 months (5% mortality in combined therapy group versus 11% in CABG-alone group). There was no significant difference in anginal class and no improvement in exercise tolerance at 12 months discernible between the two groups. Five year follow-up [6] was conducted at 13 surgical centers that had enrolled 83% (218/263) of the subjects originally. The study was conducted in 89% of the survivors (128/144) who completed the original trial. Although both groups had sustained angina improvement, the CABG plus TMR group ($n = 68$) had a significantly lower mean CCS score (0.4 ± 0.7 versus 0.7 ± 1.1) and a lower proportion of patients with severe angina (0% versus 10%) compared with the CABG-alone group ($n = 60$). In addition, the CABG/ plus TMR group trended to have higher proportion of patients that were angina-free (78% versus 63%). The Kaplan–Meier survival at 6 years was similar between both groups (76% versus 80%).

Peterson *et al.* [8] performed a comprehensive review of all TMR cases from January 1998 to December 2001 using the STS national cardiac database. The study included data from 131 institutions and 3717 TMR procedures performed in community practice. Of the 3717 patients, only 661 had TMR alone and 2475 had TMR plus CABG. The overall baseline demographics of the two groups were comparable with each other as well as with those of the published RCTs. The patients had a mean age of 62–65 years and a mean ejection fraction of 46–50%. The in-hospital mortality rate for the TMR-only group was 6.4% compared with 4.2% seen in the TMR plus CABG group. The combined rates of operative mortality rates or morbidity (defined as reoperation, prolonged ventilation, renal failure, stroke, or deep sternal wound infection) for TMR only and TMR plus CABG groups were 14.8% and 17.2%, respectively.

Of the 2475 TMR plus CABG procedures, only 390 were identified as having triple vessel disease and receiving less than three bypass grafts. This group was compared with the reported 39 454 CABG procedures in the same time frame identified with triple-vessel disease and also receiving less than three bypass grafts. The unadjusted incidence of mortality and morbidity in the TMR plus CABG group was noted to be higher than the CABG-only group (18.8% versus 15.5%) although not reaching statistical significance ($P = 0.09$). There was also a trend toward a higher mortality rate in the TMR plus CABG group (4.9% versus 4.1%) although not statistically significant ($P = 0.37$). These data fail to confirm the results of two RCTs [20,21] which reported significantly lower mortality rates in the CABG plus TMR group compared with the CABG-alone group. However, the study of Peterson *et al.* [8] has been criticized because diffuse coronary artery disease itself is likely to be an independent predictor of operative mortality and was not controlled [6]. Furthermore, it is likely that there were differences between the two groups with respect to the viability of ungrafted areas, necessarily making risk adjustment impossible [6].

There is no conclusive evidence that TMR, as an adjunct to CABG, will help increase myocardial perfusion or function of ischemic viable myocardial regions with ungraftable targets. However, based on the evidence available and in a carefully screened and appropriately selected patient population, TMR can offer possible synergistic symptomatic relief for patients who otherwise would be incompletely revascularized by traditional CABG. Future studies utilizing positron emission testing and magnetic resonance imaging offer the possibility of assessing myocardial perfusion at the tissue level and may help to elucidate the mechanism of action of TMR-based symptom relief. Further controlled, multicenter, blinded RCTs will help to clarify the apparent clinical benefits and risks of TMR as an adjunct to CABG.

References

1 Allen KB, Dowling RD, Fudge TL, *et al.* Comparison of transmyocardial revascularization with medical therapy in patients with refractory angina. *N Engl J Med* 1999;**341**: 1029–36.

2 Frazier OH, March RJ, Horvath KA. Transmyocardial revascularization with a carbon dioxide laser in patients with end-stage coronary disease. *N Engl J Med* 1999;**341**:1021–8.

3 Burkhoff D, Schmidt S, Schulman SP, *et al.* Transmyocardial revascularization compared with continued medical therapy for treatment of refractory angina pectoris: a prospective randomized trial. *Lancet* 1999;**354**:885–90.

4 Schofield PM, Sharples LD, Caine N, *et al.* Transmyocardial laser revascularization in patients with refractory angina: a randomized controlled trial. *Lancet* 1999;**353**:519–24.

5 Aaberge L, Nordstrand K, Dragsund M, *et al.* Transmyocardial revascularization with CO_2 laser in patients with refractory angina pectoris. Clinical results from the Norwegian randomized trial. *J Am Coll Cardiol* 2000;**35**:1170–7.

6 Aaberge L, Rootwelt K, Blomhoff S, *et al.* Continued symptomatic improvement three to five years after transmyocardial revascularization with CO(2) laser: a late clinical follow-up of the Norwegian randomized trial with transmyocardial revascularization. *J Am Coll Cardiol* 2002;**39**:1588–93.

7 Allen KB, Dowling RD, Schuch DR, *et al.* Adjunctive transmyocardial revascularization: five-year follow-up of a prospective, randomized trial. *Ann Thorac Surg* 2004;**78**:458–65.

8 Horvath KA, Aranki SF, Cohn LH, *et al.* Sustained angina relief 5 years after transmyocardial laser revascularization with a CO(2) laser. *Circulation* 2001;**104**(12 Suppl 1):81–4.

9 Allen KB, Dowling RD, Angell WW, *et al.* Transmyocardial revascularization: 5-year follow-up of a prospective, randomized multicenter trial. *Ann Thorac Surg* 2004;**77**:1228–34.

10 Peterson ED, Kaul P, Kaczmarek RG, *et al.* From controlled trials to clinical practice: monitoring transmyocardial revascularization use and outcomes. *J Am Coll Cardiol* 2003;**42**: 1611–6.

11 Lutter G, Martin J, von Samson P, *et al.* Microperfusion enhancement after TMLR in chronically ischemic porcine hearts. *Cardiovasc Surg* 2001;**9**:281–91.

12 Lutter G, Sarai K, Nitzsche E, *et al.* Evaluation of transmyocardial laser revascularization by following objective parameters of perfusion and ventricular function. *Thorac Cardiovasc Surg* 2000;**48**:79–85.

13 Stamou SC, Boyce SW, Cooke RH, *et al.* One-year outcome after combined coronary artery bypass grafting and transmyocardial laser revascularization for refractory angina pectoris. *Am J Cardiol* 2002;**89**:1365–8.

14 Trehan N, Mishra M, Bapna R, *et al.* Transmyocardial laser revascularisation combined with coronary artery bypass grafting without cardiopulmonary bypass. *Eur J Cardiothorac Surg* 1997;**12**:276–84.

15 Trehan N, Mishra Y, Mehta Y, *et al.* Transmyocardial laser as an adjunct to minimally invasive CABG for complete myocardial revascularization. *Ann Thorac Surg* 1998;**66**: 1113–8.

16 Gregoric I, Messner G, Couto WJ, *et al.* Off-pump coronary artery bypass grafting and transmyocardial laser revascularization via a left thoracotomy. *Texas Heart Inst J* 2003;**30**:13–8.

17 Vincent JG, Bardos P, Kruse J, *et al.* End stage coronary disease treated with the transmyocardial CO_2 laser revascularization: a chance for the 'inoperable' patient. *Eur J Cardiothorac Surg* 1997;**11**:888–94.

18 Diegeler A, Schneider J, Lauer B, *et al.* Transmyocardial laser revascularization using the holium-YAG laser for treatment of end stage coronary artery disease. *Eur J Cardiothorac Surg* 1998;**13**:392–7.

19 Wehberg KE, Julian JS, Todd JC 3rd, *et al.* Improved patient outcomes when transmyocardial revascularization is used as adjunctive revascularization. *Heart Surg Forum* 2003;**6**:328–30.

20 Allen KB, Dowling RD, DelRossi AJ, *et al.* Transmyocardial laser revascularization combined with coronary artery bypass grafting: a multicenter, blinded, prospective, randomized, controlled trial. *J Thorac Cardiovasc Surg* 2000;**119**:540–9.

21 Frazier OH, Boyce SW, Griffith BP, *et al.* Transmyocardial revascularization using a synchronized CO_2 laser as adjucnt to coronary artery bypass grafting: results of a prospective, randomized multi-center trial with 12 month follow-up. *Circulation* 1999;**100**(Suppl 1):1248.

22 Loubani M, Chin D, Leverment JN, *et al.* Mid-term results of combined transmyocardial laser revascularization and coronary artery bypass. *Ann Thorac Surg* 2003;**76**:1163–6.

CHAPTER 9

Operative techniques of transmyocardial laser revascularization

Keith A Horvath

Introduction

Transmyocardial laser revascularization (TMR) was developed to treat patients with severe angina resulting from end-stage coronary artery disease that was not amenable to revascularization by coronary artery bypass grafting (CABG) or percutaneous coronary interventions (PCI). Initially performed by Mirhoseini and Okada [1–3], TMR was used in combination with CABG in the early 1980s. The use of a laser as sole therapy on the beating heart required advancements in the technology. Two wavelengths of light have been approved for clinical use. Both carbon dioxide (CO_2) and holmium:yttrium-aluminum-garnet (Ho:YAG) were approved by the US Food and Drug Administration in the late 1990s after multiple non-randomized and randomized controlled trials from individual and multicenter studies demonstrated the significant improvement in angina relief after TMR [4–11]. These studies have demonstrated the safety and efficacy of the procedure as sole therapy for disabling angina in patients with diffuse coronary artery disease. TMR has been increasingly used in combination with CABG to provide a more complete revascularization to ungraftable territories of the heart.

The details of the aforementioned trials have been described elsewhere. The focus of this chapter is to describe the operative technique.

Background

As sole therapy, the procedure is performed on patients with severe disabling angina, the majority of whom are in Canadian Cardiovascular Society (CCS) angina class IV. By definition, these patients have recurrent chest pain that significantly alters their quality of life and is refractory to maximal medical therapy. Other surgical options for such patients are limited. For the sole-therapy patient, the possibility of cardiac transplantation exists, although most of these patients have a reasonable ejection fraction and are not suffering from heart failure as much as they are suffering from angina. Because of the scarcity of organs, these patients rarely undergo transplantation. Extensive coronary revascularization and endarterectomies may also be an option, but these procedures carry a higher rate of risk.

Of patients treated with TMR as sole therapy, 75% experience a significant reduction in angina postoperatively (i.e. decrease in angina of two or more classes). These results at 1 year have been maintained beyond 5 years [12]. In addition to the symptomatic improvement, objective findings, including the improvement in myocardial perfusion with a CO_2 laser, have also been documented. This improvement in symptoms and perfusion is achieved while the patients typically decrease their medical regimen. All this can be achieved with a morbidity and mortality that is typically less than that of a reoperative CABG. Of note, however, patients with recent or ongoing episodes of unstable angina requiring intravenous medications to control their chest pain have had a higher mortality rate because of the tenuous nature of their disease and the instability of their condition. Although such patients can undergo TMR as sole therapy, their risk is reduced if they can be stabilized and off intravenous antianginals for at least 2 weeks.

Preoperative assessment

Patients who undergo TMR as sole therapy present with severe angina that requires frequent use of sublingual nitroglycerin to carry out their activities of daily living, often leading to repeated hospital admissions. In at least one study, such patients were admitted on average five times in the year prior to undergoing TMR; as a group, these patients averaged 0.5 admissions in the year post-TMR [11]. These patients are well known to their internist and cardiologist and are on maximal medical therapy to control their symptoms. In addition to verifying the severity of their symptoms, preoperative assessment includes documentation of severe coronary artery disease, which typically includes a recent cardiac catheterization. The angiogram is worth repeating if it has not been performed in the previous 6 months. Occasionally, progression of disease in vein grafts (as many of these patients have undergone previous bypass surgery) may be amenable to conventional methods of revascularization. Once the diffuse nature of the disease is confirmed, evidence of reversible ischemia should be documented. Evidence may be obtained with myocardial perfusion scanning; rest, and stress echocardiography; or with cine and perfusion magnetic resonance imaging. The procedure should be avoided in patients in whom a very small amount of myocardial ischemia is surrounded by a significant area of myocardial infarction as the success in such patients is limited. Additionally, a severely depressed ejection fraction (<20%) was used as a cut-off point for the aforementioned clinical trials, and TMR should not be considered as therapy for heart failure unless a significant amount of reversible ischemia or hibernating myocardium is present that may lead to an improvement in myocardial function after revascularization.

Used in combination with CABG, the preoperative evaluation is the same as that of any CABG patient. The decision to use TMR in combination is frequently made intraoperatively. For example, an occluded artery on an angiogram may prove to be graftable in the operating room and may be revascularized by

CABG. If not bypassable, then the decision to use TMR would be made at that time. By review of the angiogram, the surgeon may have an idea of whether all territories will be graftable. For patients in whom TMR may be beneficial as an adjunct, its use is discussed preoperatively.

Anesthesia

TMR for sole-therapy patients is performed via a left thoracotomy, and therefore their general anesthetic can be supplemented by a thoracic epidural. This approach is beneficial in managing postoperative pain. Additionally, single-lung ventilation via bronchial blocker or double lumen endotracheal tube may assist the surgeon in exposure, particularly in patients who have had previous CABG. If an epidural is not used, then analgesia post-thoracotomy may be obtained via local infiltration of the intercostal muscle with local anesthetic. For patients who undergo TMR plus CABG, the anesthetic is the same as for those who undergo CABG alone.

Operative technique

Sole therapy transmyocardial laser revascularization performed as an open surgical procedure is typically carried out through a left anterolateral thoracotomy in the fifth intercostal space (Fig. 9.1). The patient is placed in a supine position with a roll under the left side from the shoulder to the waist to elevate the left hemithorax. Skin preparation includes at least one or both groin areas, particularly in patients with low ejection fractions or unstable angina, as they may require intraoperative placement of an intra-aortic balloon pump. After the establishment of adequate general endotracheal anesthesia, an 8–10 cm skin incision is made as shown in Fig. 9.2. Exposure of the heart through this incision can typically be achieved without division of the ribs or costal cartilages.

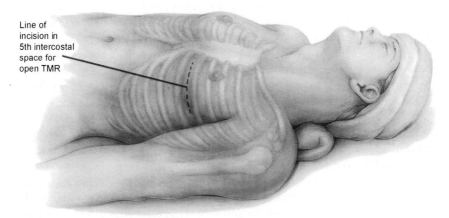

Line of incision in 5th intercostal space for open TMR

Figure 9.1 Line of incision in fifth intercostals space for open TMR.

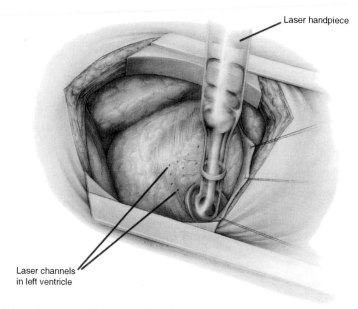

Laser handpiece

Laser channels
in left ventricle

Figure 9.2 Open transmyocardial revascularization.

Once the ribs are spread by a retractor and the lung is deflated, the pericardium is opened to expose the epicardial surface of the heart. Care must be taken to avoid previous bypass grafts. The left anterior descending artery is identified and used as a landmark of the location of the septum. The inferior and posterior lateral portions of the heart can be reached through this incision with a combination manual traction and placement of packing behind the heart and, as illustrated, the use of a right-angled laser handpiece. (The CO_2 laser uses a system of articulated arms and is delivered to the epicardial surface where a transmural channel is created with a single pulse. Ho:YAG device is delivered via a fiber and a channel is created with multiple pulses as the fiber is manually advanced through the myocardium.) Channels are created starting near the base of the heart and then serially in a line approximately 1 cm apart toward the apex, starting inferiorly and then working superiorly to the anterior surface of the heart. As some bleeding from the channels occurs, commencement of the TMR inferiorly keeps the anterior area clear and expedites the procedure. The number of channels created depends on the size of the heart and on the size of the ischemic area. Myocardium that is thinned by scar, particularly when the scar is transmural, should be avoided as TMR will be of no benefit to these regions and bleeding from channels in these areas may be problematic. Transesophageal echocardiography can be used to confirm transmural penetration of the laser energy. The vaporization of blood by the laser energy as the laser beam enters the ventricle creates an obvious and characteristic acoustic effect as noted on transesophageal echocardiography (Fig. 9.3).

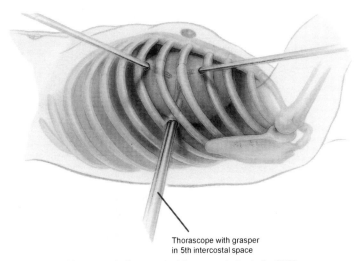

Thorascope with grasper
in 5th intercostal space

Figure 9.3 Triangulated intercostal placement of thorascopic tools for TMR.

To minimize postoperative incisional pain, particularly in patients who have not had previous bypass surgery, the TMR procedure can be performed with video-assisted thoracoscopy or robotically [13]. Again, the patient is positioned supine with the left hemithorax elevated by a roll. The left upper extremity may also be retracted cranially to facilitate placement of thoracoscope. The thoracoscopic ports may be placed in the fifth or fourth intercostal space. Through the same 10-mm port incision used for the thoracoscope, an endoscopic grasper may be placed to facilitate the dissection. Additional ports once the camera has been placed can be created under thoracoscopic guidance. As the heart is immediately adjacent to the chest wall, endoscopic instrumentation may not be necessary, and standard instruments may be introduced through these additional incisions. The incisions should be triangulated to provide maximum facility for dissection and exposure (Fig. 9.4).

This view from the thoracoscope demonstrating the grasper, which is placed through the same thoracoscope incision at 6 o'clock in Fig. 9.4, and an additional grasper placed through a third intercostal incision port at 1 o'clock. These two graspers are used to elevate and separate the pericardium, which is divided using standard dissecting scissors placed through a more anterior fifth intercostal incision. Care is taken to avoid the left phrenic nerve during this dissection.

Laser handpieces can be introduced through any of the ports with replacement of the thoracoscope as needed to allow the creation of TMR channels on all areas of the left ventricular surface. A straight handpiece, as demonstrated in Fig. 9.5, is being introduced through the third intercostal incision. With a combination of the use of the straight and right-angled handpieces, all surfaces can be

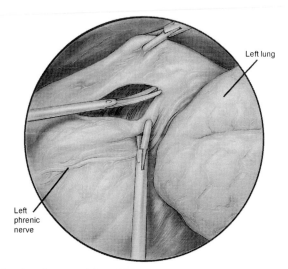

Figure 9.4 Incision of pericardium over left ventricle.

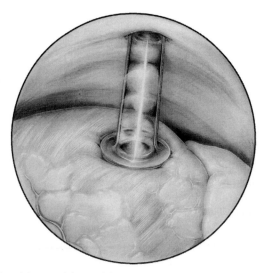

Figure 9.5 Laser handpiece on left ventricle.

covered. Bleeding from the channels is controlled either with direct finger pressure or the use of sponge stick placed after removal of the handpiece.

The thorascopic incisions are closed with three layers of absorbable suture and a dry sterile dressing is applied. A chest tube is placed through one of the fifth intercostal incision sites to provide adequate evacuation of air and/or fluid from the pleural cavity postoperatively (Fig. 9.6).

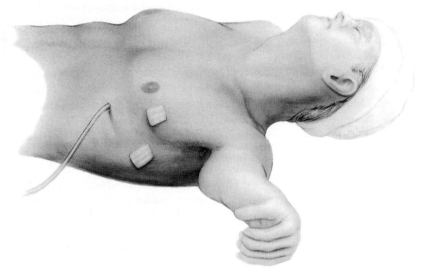

Figure 9.6 Procedure completed with closure and drainage of thoracic wounds.

Postoperative care

The majority of sole-therapy patients are extubated in the operating room. Because of the angiogenic effects, revascularization by TMR improves with time, so postoperative care is different to that of a CABG patient. Care must be taken to avoid myocardial stress, which includes adequate pain control and maintenance of perfusion pressure. Hemodynamic instability or marginal cardiac output should be treated first by insertion of an intra-aortic balloon pump. This procedure may be performed intraoperatively before TMR in patients with low ejection fractions or unstable angina. Prophylaxis for arrhythmias with a CO_2 laser is not usually required postoperatively. For TMR plus CABG, postoperative care is as for CABG alone.

Outcome

Because of the severity of their disease, sole-therapy TMR patients experience an early morbidity and mortality rate similar to that of reoperative CABG. Occasionally, chest pain may occur postoperatively, but this pain is typically less frequent than that which the patient experienced preoperatively. These symptoms typically decrease over time. Both randomized and non-randomized data indicate that 75% of patients have a decrease of two or more angina classes at 1-year follow-up. Longer term angina relief of over 5 years postoperatively has also been demonstrated with CO_2 TMR. In a recent report, patients had an average angina class of 3.7 preoperatively and the average was 1.5 at 1 year and 1.6 at 5 years postoperatively [12].

Anecdotal reports of reoperative TMR for patients who develop a new area of reversible ischemia, typically over a year after the original procedure, have been published. Some patients have undergone bypass surgery or angioplasty after TMR because of progression of their disease. As a result, recurrent chest pain late after TMR should be initially investigated with repeat cardiac catheterization to determine whether conventional methods are feasible.

The outcomes in patients who have TMR in combination with CABG have, not surprisingly, demonstrated a similar improvement in symptoms. Using cine MRI, we have demonstrated an improvement in wall motion in areas that received the laser treatment alone. Obviously, this improvement may be related to the bypass grafting for these combination patients; however, there is no evidence of microinfarction in the laser-treated areas. Further studies to delineate the benefit of TMR with CABG are underway.

For patients with severe angina resulting from diffuse coronary disease, TMR has provided significant short- and long-term angina relief. In combination with CABG, TMR also provides a method to completely revascularize patients who have both graftable and ungraftable vessels.

References

1 Mirhoseini M, Cayton MM. Revascularization of the heart by laser. *J Microsurg* 1981;**2**:253–60.

2 Mirhoseini M, Shelgikar S, Cayton MM. New concepts in revascularization of the myocardium. *Ann Thorac Surg* 1988;**45**:415–20.

3 Okada M, Ikuta H, Shimizu K, Horii H, Nakamura K. Alternate method of myocardial revascularization by laser: experimental and clinical study. *Kobe J Med Sci* 1986;**32**:151–61.

4 Horvath KA, Cohn LH, Cooley DA, et al. Transmyocardial laser revascularization: results of a multicenter trial with transmyocardial laser revascularization used as sole therapy for end-stage coronary artery disease. *J Thorac Cardiovasc Surg* 1997;**113**:645–53.

5 Schofield PM, Sharples LD, Caine N, et al. Transmyocardial laser revascularization in patients with refractory angina: a randomized controlled trial. *Lancet* 1999;**353**:519–24.

6 Cooley DA, Frazier OH, Kadipasaoglu KA, et al. Transmyocardial laser revascularization: clinical experience with twelve-month follow-up. *J Thorac Cardiovasc Surg* 1996;**111**:791–9.

7 Frazier OH, Cooley DA, Kadipasaoglu KA, et al. Myocardial revascularization with laser: preliminary findings. *Circulation* 1995;**92**(Suppl 2):58–65.

8 Horvath KA, Mannting F, Cummings N, Sherman SK, Cohn LH. Transmyocardial laser revascularization: operative techniques and clinical results at two years. *J Thorac Cardiovasc Surg* 1996;**111**:1047–53.

9 Allen KB, Dowling RD, Fudge TL, et al. Comparison of transmyocardial revascularization with medical therapy in patients with refractory angina. *N Engl J Med* 1999;**341**:1029–36.

10 Burkhoff D, Schmidt S, Schulman SP, et al. Transmyocardial laser revascularization compared with continued medical therapy for treatment of refractory angina pectoris: a prospective randomized trial. *Lancet* 1999;**354**:885–90.

11 Frazier OH, March RJ, Horvath KA. Transmyocardial revascularization with a carbon dioxide laser in patients with end-stage coronary artery disease. *N Engl J Med* 1999;**341**:1021–8.

12 Horvath KA, Aranki SF, Cohn LH, *et al.* Sustained angina relief 5 years after transmyocardial laser revascularization with CO_2 laser. *Circulation* 2001;**104**(Suppl 1):81–4.

13 Horvath KA. Thoracoscopic transmyocardial laser revascularization. *Ann Thorac Surg* 1998;**65**:1439–41.

CHAPTER 10

The open channel hypothesis for transmyocardial revascularization: a re-examination

Peter Whittaker and Chad E Darling

Introduction

The question of whether or not blood can flow from the ventricular lumen through man-made channels and into the surrounding myocardium has, for the apparent majority of investigators, been answered in the negative. This conclusion is not unreasonably based on the near universal finding that the channels become occluded, first by thrombus and coagulated protein and later by scar tissue [1–3]. Such channel closure has been found by many investigators using many different devices in many different animal models, including human subjects, and is documented in detail elsewhere in the book. Therefore, the search for a mechanism to explain the positive clinical effects of transmyocardial revascularization (TMR) has moved on to other topics, and a chapter discussing blood flow through open channels might be expected to be brief. In fact, most current reviews of the subject devote little space to the concept of open channels and frequently contain statements similar to the following by Paul *et al.* [4], "With this body of evidence, the channel theory has largely been discounted." Other investigators have been more emphatic and have stated that, "on the basis of all these data and the theoretical arguments against it, the direct blood flow hypothesis must be rejected" [5]. Nevertheless, the failure to pinpoint the mechanism of TMR's clinical benefit despite the extensive investigation of several alternatives to channel-derived blood flow, combined with evidence that some channels are indeed open months after the procedure, may indicate that the "open channel theory" should not yet be completely rejected. The original intent, as obviously implied by the name, was for TMR to revascularize hypoperfused tissue and hence restore an adequate blood supply. Therefore, in this chapter we consider the primary requirements for establishing and documenting revascularization; specifically:

1 the presence of open channels;
2 the opportunity for blood flow through such channels;
3 methods of flow detection; and
4 whether channel flow could be sufficient to be of clinical benefit.

Open channels – is there any histologic evidence?

In stark contrast to the overwhelming majority of both animal and human studies that have reported closed channels, there are a very small number of published reports of open channels. In rat hearts, we found that channels made using an ultraviolet laser (a frequency-tripled neodymium:YAG laser; wavelength 355 nm) were open at the end of the protocol; 51–165 days after they were originally made [6]. In this study, the channels were made using 400 and 600 μm diameter optic fibers; however, at the end of the protocol, the average channel width was approximately 35 μm (the largest was 140 μm). In a similar study, we found that channels made using a 25-gauge hypodermic syringe needle, with an external diameter of 400 μm, had a maximum width of 40 μm when examined 2 months later [7]. In both studies, we observed vascular connections to the channels and confirmed, through serial sectioning, that the open spaces observed did connect to the ventricular lumen and thus were actual channels rather than the channel remnants that have been reported in some studies. In all of these cases, the open channels were surrounded by bands of fibrosis, which were usually much wider than the channels themselves (Fig. 10.1). Open channels, or at least remnants of open channels (connection to the ventricular cavity was not confirmed), were also found in sheep hearts 30 days after ultraviolet laser TMR (wavelength 308 nm) [8]. There may be a potential correlation between channel patency and the wavelength of the laser used and, perhaps more importantly, the amount and type of injury produced when the channel is made [9]; however, this possibility has not been systematically examined.

There is no question that despite the potential advantages of using three-dimensional reconstruction methods to confirm potential channel–lumen connections [10], conventional two-dimensional histologic analysis has been

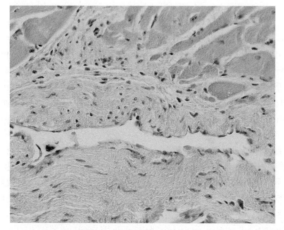

Figure 10.1 Open channel (approximately 20 μm wide) in rat heart 3 months after it was made using an ultraviolet laser (wavelength 308 nm). Serial sectioning demonstrated that the channel connected to the left ventricular cavity. Hematoxylin and eosin stain.

almost exclusively used and appears to have been adequate to demonstrate that open channels are rarely seen in human hearts. On the other hand, despite the more than 10 000 cases that have now been performed, there are very few published histology reports. Furthermore, none of these studies present data from more than 10 patients (indeed many are single case reports) and most have examined tissue from patients who died soon after surgery or who subsequently underwent heart transplantation and hence cannot be considered to represent successful examples of TMR. In the three largest series (10, 8, and 4 patients, respectively), tissue from all but one patient was examined 20 or fewer days after TMR surgery [11,12,1]. No connections were found between the left ventricular cavity and open channels in any of these hearts, which were all treated with carbon dioxide lasers. At least some of these patients were identified as having derived no clinical benefit from TMR (i.e., there was no reduction in angina pain); however, such an association has not been found in every case. For example, Summers *et al.* [13] examined a heart from a 60-year-old man, who had severe angina pectoris (Canadian Cardiovascular Society class IV) prior to surgery, but was asymptomatic when evaluated 3 and 6 months later. Approximately 9 months after surgery, he died in a motor vehicle accident. Numerous focal scars aligned approximately perpendicular to the epicardial surface were found; however, no open channels were seen. In contrast, the Texas Heart Institute group described findings from a patient who died of coronary artery disease-related causes 3 months after carbon dioxide laser TMR surgery [14]. In the original surgery, 25 of 30 applied laser pulses were confirmed by transesophageal echocardiography to have penetrated the entire thickness of the wall. Regions of the heart containing endocardial indentations were sectioned and nine endothelial-lined channels aligned perpendicular to the epicardial surface were identified. Direct connections between some of these channels and both the ventricular lumen and intramyocardial blood vessels were seen; however, the channels were small, 20–75 μm wide, and, as with the open channels seen in animal hearts, they were also surrounded by wide bands of fibrosis (150–500 μm). Mirhoseini's original laser TMR papers [15] also contain illustrations of supposed open channels in human hearts observed more than 1 year after TMR and following cancer-related (i.e., not cardiovascular) death. Nonetheless, it is difficult to state unequivocally that the structures shown are actual laser channels. The relationship between the channels and the endocardial surface is not described and cannot be seen from the high-magnification micrographs. In addition, in contrast to most examples, there is very little fibrosis surrounding the channels. Another study identified channel remnants, approximately 1 mm in diameter (direct connections to the left ventricular cavity were not claimed), in the heart of a patient 6 months after TMR, at which time the patient received a heart transplant because of recurrent angina pectoris and progressive heart failure [16]. Unfortunately, the laser used in this particular study cannot be identified – the manufacturer is listed as "PLC Eclipse Surgical Technologies" (sic).

In the search for laser channels, it should be recognized that there are natural structures, thebesian vessels, that could be mistaken for open channels. These conduits, which drain directly into the ventricular lumen, were discovered in the early 18th century; however, consideration of their potential role in the 21st century practice of TMR has been limited to only a couple of papers. Ansari [17] examined sheep hearts, *ex vivo*, for the presence of thebesian vessels specifically because this animal has been used in TMR experiments. India ink was injected into the coronary sinus, the right coronary artery, or the left coronary artery after ligation of the coronary veins, and the endocardial surface was examined for the presence of ink and ink-filled vessels. Although the number of direct ventricular connections found was relatively small (no more than 10 in a single ventricle) and were more commonly located in the right rather than the left ventricle, they were present in all but one of the 36 hearts examined. In both ventricles, the vessels were found predominantly in the apical region and at the base of the papillary muscles. In addition, the majority of the connections appeared to be venoluminal (i.e., between venules and the ventricular chamber) rather than arterioluminal or from capillary drainage. Histologically, only the arterioluminal vessels contained smooth muscle, while the endothelial cell lined venoluminal vessels were very thin walled. Micrographs of the latter structures appear quite similar to that illustrated in the some of the "laser channels" shown in Mirhoseini's work [15]. The presence of thebesian vessels in human hearts is well documented [18,19] and should therefore be considered when histology from TMR cases is examined.

Open channels alone are not enough for TMR to be effective in revascularization and, for any blood flow to be useful, there must be communication between the channels and the myocardium. In the original premise for TMR, based on blood flow in the highly trabeculated structure of reptilian hearts, the channels communicated with sinusoids. Without doubt, sinusoids are common in reptile [20] and fish hearts [21] and can also be found in humans; however, in the latter, they represent a rare pathology usually associated with early death or the need for transplant [22,23]. Thus, the lack of trabeculation and sinusoids in normal human hearts [24] means that open channel–myocardium communication would have to occur through vascular connections. Again, support for the existence of such connections is limited to only a few reports as described earlier. One additional piece of supporting evidence that has seldom been referenced comes from the first clinical trial of laser TMR conducted at the San Francisco Heart Institute by Crew [25]. One patient, who experienced a three-class reduction on the Canadian Cardiovascular Society scale after TMR surgery, died of a stroke 6 months later. After the heart had been fixed in formalin, Mercox, a synthetic resin, was infused into the left ventricular chamber, allowed to harden, and then the myocardium was dissolved with concentrated sodium and potassium hydroxide solutions. The resulting vascular corrosion cast revealed patent channels connecting to other vascular structures within the heart [25].

It is surprising, particularly given the lack of an established mechanism of action for TMR, that more histologic study of human tissue has not been performed. Certainly, with many of the patients referred to the surgical centers performing TMR coming from other locations and sometimes even other countries, follow-up and the collection of tissue samples from necropsy is undoubtedly challenging. However, it would also be difficult and perhaps unwise to draw conclusions based on an analysis of only a fraction of 1% of the total number of treated patients. In addition, it could be argued that most of the patients who have died represent a subpopulation in whom TMR was not as successful as it presumably was in those patients who are still alive. Specifically, it is possible that long-term survival may be associated with the presence of open channels.

In conclusion, there is convincing histologic evidence to support the notion that, in some instances, channels made in human and animal hearts can be open months after they are made, and that such open channels can connect to both the left ventricular cavity and the myocardial vasculature. Nevertheless, there are very few studies to have documented such findings and the preponderance of evidence, at least from animal studies, indicates that the vast majority of channels are closed. Nevertheless, there are potential explanations for why channel making in humans could produce different results from the animal experiments (e.g., the larger amount of fibrosis in diseased human hearts than in healthy animal hearts could limit the extent of thermal injury [26]). Therefore, the relative dearth of human studies still allows the possibility that open channels occur more frequently than is currently believed.

Is flow through open channels possible?

Soon after the initial reports of myocardial channel creation using needles appeared in the 1950s, Pifarré et al. [27] pointed out a potentially major flaw in the concept; because the intramyocardial pressure exceeded that within the ventricular cavity throughout the cardiac cycle, then blood flow through the channels was a "physiologic impossibility." Since that time, although the methods used to measure intramyocardial pressure have been refined and improved, several studies have confirmed Pifarré's original contention that intramyocardial wall pressure exceeds ventricular cavity pressure [28,29]. Indeed, when invited to revisit his original publication 30 years later in response to the advent of laser-based TMR, he saw no reason to revise his opinion [30]. Nonetheless, measurement of intramyocardial pressure is not a trivial matter. For example, although Kingma et al. [31] found that the pressure values obtained using solid-state Millar and Konigsberg micromanometric transducers in non-ischemic canine hearts exceeded those in the left ventricular cavity in both systole and diastole, the measurements did depend upon the orientation of the sensors with respect to the left ventricular cavity, the type of transducer used, and that the magnitude of this difference varied with insertion depth (subepicardial values exhibited the largest intersensor difference). Of note, the pressure difference between the subendocardial tissue and the left ventricular cavity in diastole was 5.0 ± 2.4 mmHg ($P = 0.04$) measured using the Millar transducer, but was only 2.2 ± 2.4 mmHg using the Konigsberg transducer ($P = $ NS), which may even provide for the possibility of a limited amount of diastolic flow.

In contrast, one recent study, in isolated working pig hearts, suggested that during periods of ischemia, intramyocardial pressure falls below ventricular pressure, measured using a Millar transducer, at end-systole [32] and hence the pressure gradient would not prevent flow into an open channel. Nevertheless, the pressure gradient in favor of channel flow was less than 5 mmHg and the duration of this opportunity was less than 0.05 s. Thus, the amount of flow that could be delivered under these circumstances would be extremely limited.

Although such results and arguments appear difficult to refute, anyone who has ever performed TMR or has seen TMR knows, without any shadow of a doubt, that blood can indeed flow vigorously from the ventricular cavity into the laser-made channels and then spurt out of the heart. This apparent paradox is difficult to reconcile. Some have argued that the left ventricular cavity to atmospheric pressure gradient may be the one that permits flow to exit through the channels; however, it would still appear that if the pressure within the ventricular wall exceeds that of the blood pressure, then flow would not occur. Nevertheless, there is also no doubt that the mechanics of myocardial contraction and flow within the tissue are complex, involving changes not only in the material properties of myocardium during contraction, but also in wall stretch and ventricular pressure [33]. The difficulties in obtaining accurate measurements of intramyocardial pressure combined with our incomplete knowledge of the relationship between ventricular mechanics and flow within the wall suggest that the best available evidence is that the practical experience of seeing flow through the channels immediately after they are made indicates that under certain circumstances flow can indeed occur.

Can flow through channels be detected?

If the channels were open and if blood did flow through them, would it be possible to detect that flow? One provocative TMR study provides evidence not only to support the two conditional clauses, but also that the answer to the question could be yes. Reuthebuch *et al.* [34] used myocardial contrast echocardiography (MCE) in an attempt to image flow through laser channels. In 15 patients, examined 2–3 months after an average of 20 transmural channels were made using a carbon dioxide laser (some patients also received bypass grafts), 6 mL contrast medium was injected via a catheter directly into the left ventricular cavity. Even though coronary angiography and ventriculography revealed no patent channels in any of the patients, MCE detected the passage of contrast medium into one or two (1.5 ± 0.5) myocardial "channels", located in the apical region, in 10 patients. The entry of contrast medium into the ventricular wall occurred only during systole and was seen to a penetration depth of 0.7 ± 0.1 cm, with an eventual lateral spread from the initial location of 1.4 ± 0.4 cm. Conversely, when contrast medium was injected into the coronary arteries or into bypass grafts, it did not drain into the left ventricular cavity through the channels. The failure to detect similar channels in five additional patients, who had bypass graft surgery but not TMR, prompted the authors to conclude that the imaged structures were not thebesian vessels. Nevertheless, MCE has been used to demonstrate thebesian vein outflow in human hearts [35]. An evaluation of 29 patients (27 with coronary artery disease and two with hypertrophic cardiomyopathy) revealed the presence of contrast medium within the ventricular cavity after injection into the left main coronary artery in 10 subjects. The investigators reported "outflow jets" originating from the endocardial surface of the apex, anterolateral wall, and interventricular septum during end-systole in the coronary artery disease patients and during early systole in the hypertrophic cardiomyopathy patients. The variable occurrence of thebesian vessels in human hearts indicated by this study also suggests that the number of cases evaluated by Reuthebuch *et al.* to rule out the possibility that the imaged structures were thebesian vessels rather than laser channels was too small to be definitive. Thus, as with most aspects of TMR, the data are not definitive but instead provide provocative circumstantial evidence to support the use of TMR.

One acute study in sheep provides some support for the ability of MCE to detect channel-related perfusion [36]. An echo-contrast agent was injected into the left atrium soon after 15–30 transmural channels had been made using a holmium:YAG laser in five hearts. In contrast to the human study, the epicardial echocardiography used in this open-chest preparation did not reveal individual channels, but did show an "echo blush" in the region where the channels had been made, spreading from the subendocardium to the subepicardium. This change in echogenicity appeared simultaneously with the appearance of contrast in the ventricular cavity and before a faint general opacification of the ventricular wall derived from antegrade flow through the coronary arteries and so seems consistent with perfusion through the channels. The authors proposed that this technique could be used during surgery to delineate the area treated by the laser [36].

Although Reuthebuch *et al.* [34] failed to detect open channels using coronary angiography several months after TMR, angiographic images of open channels immediately after percutaneous laser myocardial revascularization have been published. For example, in a case report, Colombo *et al.* [37] observed three open channels when ventricular angiography was performed immediately after 10 channels had been made using a holmium:YAG laser. At least one of the channels was transmural and a slight pericardial effusion of the contrast agent could be seen (also suggesting that the intramyocardial–ventricular cavity pressure gradient does not preclude flow). Six months after treatment, when the patient had reported a worsening of his effort-induced chest pain, the channels were no longer visible. The authors stated that although they routinely perform left ventricular angiography immediately after laser treatment, the angiograms usually fail to confirm the presence of channels. They speculated that this failure occurred because the tip of the fiberoptic was seldom in good contact with the endocardial surface and hence channels were rarely created using the percutaneous approach [37]. Nevertheless, Perin *et al.* [38] demonstrated in a case report three open channels in an angiogram obtained immediately after percutaneous holmium:YAG treatment.

Table 10.1 Spatial resolution of imaging methods and their advantages and disadvantages.

Imaging method	Resolution	Advantages/disadvantages
Conventional coronary angiography	~150 μm	Widely available, not optimized to visualize TMR channels, invasive, X-ray exposure
Contrast echocardiography	10 μm	Echo contrast offers best current spatial resolution, no X-ray exposure or iodinated contrast required
Single photon emission computed tomography	~ 1 cm	Limited spatial resolution, provides qualitative metabolic information
Positron emission tomography	0.3–1 cm	Limited availability, tracer uptake can provide metabolic information and quantify blood flow
Magnetic resonance imaging	~1 mm	Good spatial resolution, technology under development
Multi-row detector spiral computed tomography	~0.6 mm	Technology under development, requires contrast injection, X-ray exposure
Electron beam computed tomography	~0.8 mm	Technology under development, requires contrast injection, X-ray exposure

Table 10.1 shows the spatial resolution of several possible imaging methods in addition to some potential advantages and disadvantages (the resolution values given are an approximation derived from multiple published sources). It is clear from both Table 10.1 and the preceding discussion that because the channels are no more than 1 mm in diameter immediately after they are made and that they subsequently decrease in diameter, only coronary angiography and myocardial contrast echocardiography currently appear to have the capability to detect channel flow directly. As far as we are aware, no other imaging methods have detected TMR channels *in vivo*. Nevertheless, it is the other listed methods that have been most often employed in the search for TMR-induced perfusion changes.

Single photon emission computed tomography (SPECT) has a spatial resolution of approximately 1 cm, while that of positron emission tomography (PET) is 0.3–1 cm and so neither is able to show flow within a channel directly. Nonetheless, they are powerful methods to assess regional changes in myocardial blood flow in addition to their capacity to evaluate muscle viability and metabolism and so are the most commonly used techniques to appraise clinical outcome after TMR. Both methods require the uptake of tracers into the myocardium and therefore they are able, indirectly, to provide information regarding perfusion around channels. Thus, when used in TMR studies, hearts have been imaged before and after laser treatment to determine if regional blood flow and metabolism are enhanced in the areas where channels were placed. Despite the relatively low spatial resolution of these methods, there are some results from clinical studies that could be interpreted as being inconsistent with flow through open channels. For example, evidence from our group revealed that a large lateral wall perfusion defect seen using three-dimensional reconstruction of SPECT images obtained at stress had decreased in size from the outside edges of the defect at 6 months after TMR [39]. If there had been blood flow through laser channels, then we might have expected to see "hot-spots" denoting regions of increased flow within the perfusion defect. The observed pattern of decrease in the defect, however, appears more consistent with an in-growth of blood vessels from normally perfused tissue than it does with the presence of open channels. Even though other studies have failed to show "hot-spots" within the laser-treated region [40], it should be noted that perfusion defects represent disparities in blood flow distribution rather than ischemia and so even if there was flow through open channels, the flow may be insufficient in magnitude to eliminate the relative disparity.

Most studies using SPECT imaging to evaluate perfusion changes after TMR employ two-dimensional slices or polar mapping techniques and the subsequent division of the ventricular wall into segments [41]. The comparison of myocardial segments with such division relies on the assumption that the same segments can be matched before and after treatment. One potential problem with this assumption is that the considerable amount of tissue shrinkage that occurs after TMR (for each channel up to a 90% volume reduction from the initial necrosis to the final scar [42]) could remodel the myocardium such that normally perfused regions are pulled, by the contraction of scar tissue, into previously underperfused segments and hence could give the false impression that blood flow has been improved.

Although PET has greater spatial resolution than SPECT, it is still insufficient to image channels directly. However, PET has been used to report an improvement in subendocardial flow after TMR [43]. The authors of the study hypothesized that because channels would occlude toward the epicardial surface but remain open in the subendocardial portion, then the ratio of subendocardial to subepicardial flow would improve. Nevertheless, without a gated image-acquisition system to compensate for heart motion, it is unlikely that the spatial resolution was sufficient to measure changes in subendocardial blood flow [44]. Another carbon dioxide TMR study used a PET system capable of greater resolution than that employed by Frazier *et al.* [43] to quantify blood flow in milliliters per minute per gram of tissue, but failed to find any increase [45].

Magnetic resonance imaging (MRI) has also been used to assess regional myocardial blood flow in a limited number of clinical and experimental TMR studies [46,47]. At present, the spatial resolution is too low to identify open channels, a task further complicated by both cardiac and respiration-induced motion. However, MRI is a rapidly evolving technology and it is not unreasonable to expect that spatial resolution will improve. Two other non-invasive techniques, electron beam tomography and multi-row detector spiral computed tomography, although not in routine use, are currently being developed and hold promise for future application to TMR [48,49].

It should be noted that a potential disadvantage of the current methods for visualizing myocardial circulation is that they have been developed primarily to image flow that occurs in the conventional manner; that is, through the large epicardial arteries and their major branches. As a result, these approaches are neither designed nor optimized to detect flow in the "opposite direction" from the ventricular chamber into channels. For example, patent TMR channels would be perfused via the myocardium requiring contrast injection directly into the ventricular cavity for visualization rather than into the coronary arteries themselves.

In conclusion, limited spatial resolution precludes most of the currently available methods from directly detecting flow in narrow channels. Although methods such as SPECT, PET, and MRI are capable of detecting and even quantifying increases in regional myocardial blood flow after TMR, they cannot discern the source of the increase. The apparent ability of myocardial contrast echocardiography to detect flow in open channels indicates that additional studies to confirm or refute this finding should be undertaken.

Would flow through channels make a difference?

The preceding sections suggest that even if there is blood flow through open channels, then the amount of that flow is likely to be limited. Nevertheless, the areas that are "revascularized" by TMR had sufficient blood flow prior to surgery for the muscle cells to survive, but not enough to prevent ischemia on exertion. Thus, the key question is how much additional flow is required to eliminate the exertion deficit?

One important factor to take into account when considering this question is the ratio of oxygen supply to demand. After the creation of 30–40 channels in human hearts, quite a large amount of muscle has been vaporized or coagulated and hence the supply : demand ratio may have been favorably altered simply by reducing muscle volume and thus demand. For example, based on the assumption of a circular 1-mm diameter channel surrounded by a 1-mm circular band of muscle necrosis (total diameter of channel + necrosis = 3 mm), a wall thickness of 2 cm and 35 channels, the volume of muscle lost will be $35 \times 2(\pi d^2)/4 = 4.95$ cm^3. The usual epicardial channel spacing of 1 cm yields an approximate treated tissue volume of 48 cm^3 ($6 \times 4 \times 2$ cm). Thus, 10% of the muscle has been removed, which means a 10% increase in blood flow for the surviving muscle. Higher values for the combined diameter of channel diameter and necrosis have been reported. Lutter *et al.* [50] described a total diameter of 3–6 mm after TMR with a carbon dioxide laser – at 6 mm, the volume of muscle lost would be almost 20 cm^3, resulting in a 40% "increase" in blood flow. Therefore, even a small amount of flow through the channels may have a greater than expected impact because of the necrosis-mediated reduction in demand.

Another mechanism whereby even a small increase in blood flow could have a disproportionately large effect is through the potential connection between exercise and vascular remodeling; specifically, exercise-induced angiogenesis [51] and the transformation of capillaries into aterioles [52]. If this link could be initiated, it is possible that only a small increase in blood flow could set in motion a positive circle of events; a small increase in flow permits the patient to exercise more than was possible before surgery, which then stimulates the growth of new vessels, which could in turn increase blood flow enabling more exercise and so on.

Nevertheless, it could be argued that the laser channels are too small, even when first made and prior to any healing-related diameter loss, to make a useful contribution to blood flow. Walter [53] suggested that this was indeed the case and drew attention to his own work from the 1970s in which a cannula was used to remove cylinders of myocardial tissue approximately 4 mm in diameter [54]. Positive results, specifically increased blood flow, were found when this technique was used in both acute and chronic animal studies. In contrast, there was no increase in flow if channels approximately 1 mm in diameter were made. Such large-diameter channels have not, to our knowledge, been evaluated since these reports were published. Nevertheless, a mathematical model of oxygen transport from open channels supports the concept that larger diameter channels would be more effective than the 1 mm typically used [55].

In summary, although we do not know exactly how much additional blood flow is necessary to exert a positive effect, there are some reasons to believe that even a small amount may elicit a meaningful augmentation of tissue perfusion.

Conclusions

Much of our discussion, particularly that attempting to provide support for the existence of open channels and for the demonstration of blood flow through those channels, has had to be based on results and images obtained from "provocative" case reports rather than on substantive and definitive data obtained from studies of large patient populations. Unfortunately, "provocative", rather than "substantive" and "definitive", is a word frequently associated with TMR. That such an association remains after more than 15 years and 10 000 patients is troubling and therefore it is not surprising that laser revascularization, in its various formats, has attracted much editorial scorn [56,57]. Nevertheless, our examination of the literature suggests that the possibility of blood flow through laser-made channels cannot yet be completely ruled out. Although there are considerable logistical problems involved in obtaining laser-treated hearts postmortem for histologic examination, we propose that examination of hearts from TMR patients who have survived for many years after surgery could be crucial in resolving the "open channel" hypothesis in transmyocardial laser revascularization.

Acknowledgments

We thank Professor Andrew D. McCulloch, University of California, San Diego for helpful discussion and advice during the preparation of this chapter. This work was supported in part by a grant from the Worcester Foundation for Biomedical Research.

References

1 Gassler N, Wintzer H-O, Stubbe H-M, Wullbrand A, Helmchen U. Transmyocardial laser revascularization: histological features in human nonresponder myocardium. *Circulation* 1997;**95**:371–5.

2 Sigel JE, Abramovich CM, Lytle BW, Ratliff NB. Transmyocardial laser revascularization: three sequential autopsy cases. *J Thorac Cardiovasc Surg* 1998;**115**:1381–5.

3 Burkhoff D, Fisher PE, Apfelbaum M, *et al*. Histologic evidence of transmyocardial laser channels after 4_ weeks. *Ann Thorac Surg* 1996;**61**:1532–5.

4 Paul S, Nathan M, Byrne JG, Aranki SF. Transmyocardial laser revascularization. *J Cardio-thorac Vasc Anesth* 2004;**18**:85–92.

5 Bridges CR. Myocardial laser revascularization: the controversy and the data. *Ann Thorac Surg* 2000;**69**:655–62.

6 Whittaker P, Spariosu K, Ho ZZ. Success of transmyocardial laser revascularization is determined by the amount and organization of scar tissue produced in response to initial injury: results of ultraviolet laser treatment. *Lasers Surg Med* 1999;**24**:253–60.

7 Whittaker P, Rakusan K, Kloner RA. Transmural channels can protect ischemic tissue: assessment of long-term myocardial response to laser- and needle-made channels. *Circulation* 1996;**93**:143–52.

8 Mack CA, Magovern CJ, Hahn RT, *et al*. Channel patency and neovascularization after transmyocardial revascularization using an excimer laser: results and comparisons to nonlased channels. *Circulation* 1997;**96**(Suppl 2):65–9.

9 Whittaker P. Transmyocardial revascularization: from simplicity to complexity. *Int J Cardiovasc Med Sci* 2000;**3**:33–7.

10 Schweitzer W, Maass D, Schaepman M, *et al*. Digital 3D image reconstruction of ventriculo-capillary communication as revealed in one case after transmyocardial laser revascularization. *Pathol Res Pract* 1998;**194**:65–71.

11 Schweitzer W, Schneider J, Maass D, Hardmeier T. Transmyokardiale Laserrevaskularisation. Histopaphologische Befunde an Laserkanälen bei 10 postoperativ verstorbenen Patienten 1 bis 18 Tage nach Behandlung mit einem CO_2-Laser. *Pathologe* 1997;**18**:374–84.

12 Krabatsch T, Schäper F, Leder C, *et al*. Histological findings after transmyocardial laser revascularization. *J Cardiovasc Surg* 1996;**11**:326–31.

13 Summers JH, Henry CA III, Roberts WC. Cardiac observations late after operative transmyocardial laser "revascularization". *Am J Cardiol* 1999;**84**:489–90.

14 Cooley DA, Frazier OH, Kadipasaoglu KA, *et al*. Transmyocardial laser revascularization: anatomic evidence of long-term channel patentcy. *Texas Heart Inst J* 1994;**21**:220–4.

15 Mirhoseini M, Shelgikar S, Cayton M. Clinical and histological evaluation of laser myocardial revascularization. *J Clin Laser Med Surg* 1990;**8**:73–8.

16 Domkowski PW, Biswas SS, Steenbergen C, Lowe JE. Histological evidence of angiogenesis 9 months after transmyocardial laser revascularization. *Circulation* 2001;**103**:469–71.

17 Ansari A. Anatomy and clinical significance of ventricular thebesian veins. *Clin Anat* 2001;**14**:102–10.

18 Taylor JR, Taylor AJ. Thebesian sinusoids: forgotten collaterals to papillary muscle. *Can J Cardiol* 2000;**16**:1391–7.

19 Coussement P, De Geest H. Multiple coronary artery – left ventricular communications: an unusual prominent thebesian system. *Acta Cardiologica* 1994;**49**:165–73.

20 Kohmoto T, Argenziano M, Yamamoto N, *et al*. Assessment of transmyocardial perfusion in alligator hearts. *Circulation* 1997;**95**:1357–9.

21 Sanchez-Quintana D, Garcia-Martinez V, Climent V, Hurle JM. Morphological analysis of the fish heart ventricle: myocardial and connective tissue architecture in teleost species. *Ann Anat* 1995;**177**:267–74.

22 Shah CP, Nagi KS, Thakur RK, Boughner DR, Xie B. Spongy left ventricular myocardium in an adult. *Texas Heart Inst J* 1998;**25**:150–1.

23 Angelini A, Melacini P, Barbero F, Thiene G. Evolutionary persistence of spongy myocardium in humans. *Circulation* 1999;**99**:2475.

24 Tsang JC-C, Chiu RC-J. The phantom of "myocardial sinusoids": a historical reappraisal. *Ann Thorac Surg* 1995;**60**:1831–5.

25 Crew JR. The first clinical TMR trial: historical perspective. In: Whittaker P, Abela GS (eds). *Direct Myocardial Revascularization: History, Methodology, Technology*. Boston, MA: Kluwer Academic Publishers, 1999: 143–54.

26 Whittaker P. Detection and assessment of laser-mediated injury in transmyocardial revascularization. *J Clin Laser Med Surg* 1997;**15**:261–7.

27 Pifarré R, Jasuja ML, Lynch RD, Neville WE. Myocardial revascularization by transmyocardial acupuncture: a physiologic impossibility. *J Thorac Cardiovasc Surg* 1969;**58**: 424–31.

28 Stein PD, Sabbah HN, Marzilli M, Blick EF. Comparison of the distribution of intramyocardial pressure across the canine left ventricular wall in the beating heart during diastole and in the arrested heart: evidence of epicardial muscle tone during diastole. *Circ Res* 1980;**47**:258–67.

29 Denys BG, Aubert AE, Ector H, Kesteloot H, De Geest H. Intramyocardial pressure in the canine heart: an experimental study. *J Thorac Cardiovasc Surg* 1985;**90**:888–95.

30 Pifarré R. TMR: is it still a physiologic impossibility? In: Whittaker P, Abela GS (eds). *Direct Myocardial Revascularization: History, Methodology, Technology*. Boston, MA: Kluwer Academic Publishers, 1999: 45–59.

31 Kingma JG Jr, Armour JA, Rouleau JR. Left ventricular intramyocardial pressure determination using two different solid-state micromanometric pressure sensors. *Can J Physiol Pharmacol* 1996;**74**:701–5.

32 Modersohn D, Eddicks S, Ast I, Holinski S, Konertz W. Influence of transmyocardial laser revascularization (TMLR) on regional cardiac function and metabolism in an isolated hemoperfused working pig heart. *Int J Artif Organs* 2002;**25**:1074–81.

33 Vis MA, Bovendeerd PHM, Sipkema P, Westerhof N. Effect of ventricular contraction, pressure, and wall stretch on vessels at different locations in the wall. *Am J Physiol* 1997;**272**:H2963–75.

34 Reuthebuch O, Berwing K, Roth M, Klövekorn W-P, Bauer EP. Contrast-echocardiography: confirmation of patency of laser channels after transmyocardial laser revascularization. *Eur J Echocardiogr* 2002;**3**:24–31.

35 Cornel JH, Ten Cate FJ, Serruys PW. Myocardial contrast echocardiography can depict thebesian vein outflow in humans. *Am Heart J* 1992;**123**:1373–4.

36 Choo SJ, Shah PM, Oury JH, Duran CMG. Contrast echocardiography as an intraoperative method to determine the area of myocardium perfused by transmyocardial laser channels: an experimental study. *J Cardiovasc Surg* 1998;**13**:484–8.

37 Colombo A, Danna P, Viecca M. Angiographic evidence of myocardial channels after percutaneous transmyocardial laser treatment. *Ital Heart J* 2002;**3**:532–3.

38 Perin EC, Dohmann HJF, Dohmann HFR, de Mattos NDSG, Carvalho LA. Laser channels after precutaneous transmyocardial revascularization. *Circulation* 1999;**99**:2218.

39 Kavanagh GJ, Whittaker P, Prejean CA Jr, *et al*. Dissociation between improvement in angina pectoris and myocardial perfusion after transmyocardial revascularization with an excimer laser. *Am J Cardiol* 2001;**87**:229–31.

40 Grüning T, Kropp J, Wiener S, *et al*. Evaluation of transmyocardial laser revascularization (TMLR) by gated myocardial perfusion scintigraphy. *Ann Nucl Med* 1999;**13**:361–6.

41 Horvath KA, Cohn LH, Cooley DA, *et al*. Transmyocardial laser revascularization: results of a multicenter trial with transmyocardial laser revascularization used as sole therapy for end-stage coronary artery disease. *J Thorac Cardiovasc Surg* 1997;**113**:645–54.

42 Fisher PE, Khomoto T, DeRosa CM, *et al*. Histologic analysis of transmyocardial channels: comparison of CO_2 and holmium:YAG lasers. *Ann Thorac Surg* 1997;**64**:466–72.

43 Frazier OH, Cooley DA, Kadipasaoglu KA, *et al*. Myocardial revascularization with laser: preliminary findings. *Circulation* 1995;**92**(Suppl 2):58–65.

44 Schöder H, Schelbert HR. Nuclear imaging techniques for evaluation of TMLR. In: Whittaker P, Abela GS (eds). *Direct Myocardial Revascularization: History, Methodology, Technology*. Boston, MA: Kluwer Academic Publishers, 1999: 163–78.

45 Rimoldi O, Burns SM, Rosen SD, *et al*. Measurement of myocardial blood flow with positron emission tomography before and after transmyocardial laser revascularization. *Circulation* 1999;**100**(Suppl 2):134–8.

46 Laham RJ, Simons M, Pearlman JD, Ho KKL, Baim DS. Magnetic resonance imaging demonstrates improved regional systolic wall motion and thickening and myocardial perfusion of myocardial territories treated by laser myocardial revascularization. *J Am Coll Cardiol* 2002;**39**:1–8.

47 Mühling OM, Wang Y, Panse P, *et al*. Transmyocardial laser revascularization preserves regional myocardial perfusion: an MRI first pass perfusion study. *Cardiovasc Res* 2003;**57**:63–70.

48 Nieman K, van Geuns R-JM, Wielopolski P, Pattynama PMT, de Feyter PJ. Noninvasive coronary imaging in the new millennium: a comparison of computed tomography and magnetic resonance techniques. *Rev Cardiovasc Med* 2002;**3**:77–84.

49 Budoff MJ, Achenbach S, Duerinckx A. Clinical utility of computed tomography and magnetic resonance techniques for noninvasive coronary angiography. *J Am Coll Cardiol* 2003;**42**:1867–78.

50 Lutter G, Schwarzkopf J, Lutz C, Martin J, Beyersdorf F. Histologic findings of transmyocardial laser channels after two hours. *Ann Thorac Surg* 1998;**65**:1437–9.

51 Przyklenk K, Groom AC. Effects of exercise frequency, intensity, and duration on revascularization in the transition zone of infarcted rat hearts. *Can J Physiol Pharmacol* 1985;**63**:273–8.

52 Brown MD. Exercise and coronary vascular remodeling in the healthy heart. *Exp Physiol* 2003;**88**:645–58.

53 Walter PJ. Are the channels too small in transmyocardial laser revascularization? *Texas Heart Inst J* 2002;**29**:154.

54 Walter P, Lamprecht W, Hundeshagen H, Borst HG. Myocardial blood flow and alterations of LDH isoenzymes in infarcted heart muscle and after transmural punctures. *Cardiology* 1971;**56**:371–6.

55 Waters SL. A mathematical model for the laser treatment of heart disease. *J Biomech* 2204;**37**:281–8.

56 Schwartz Y. LMR: time to end the saga. *Cardiac Vasc Regen* 2000;**1**:214–5.

57 Turi ZG. Guided laser myocardial revascularization with coronary angioplasty: the emperor shops for new clothes. *Catheter Cardiovasc Interv* 2001;**53**:241–2.

CHAPTER 11

Mechanisms of TMR: angiogenesis

Marc P Pelletier, Varun Kapila, and Ray CJ Chiu

Historical perspective

In 1965, Sen devised an operation aimed at utilizing intraventricular blood to oxygenate the myocardial tissue through holes created with a 19-gauge needle. Contrary to normal coronary perfusion, the myocardium could then receive oxygenated blood during systole and this could occur regardless of the state of the patient's coronary anatomy. His studies showed that transmyocardial revascularization (TMR) was able to reduce infarct size and mortality in dogs following ligation of the left anterior descending artery (LAD) [1,2]. Sen had also demonstrated histologic evidence of patent transmural channels several weeks after their creation. By the early 1970s, coronary artery bypass grafting (CABG) became the most effective and preferred method of revascularization, although patients with diffuse coronary occlusive disease and those whose coronary artery disease continue to progress despite numerous re-operations could not benefit from such direct revascularization procedures. The idea of TMR was rejuvenated in the early 1980s by Mihroseini, who was the first to report on an experiment using CO_2 laser to create transmyocardial channels [3]. Mainly from his work, it was believed that the beneficial effects of TMR stemmed from its ability to create patent channels through which blood flow to the myocardium could be restored despite occluded coronary arteries (Table 11.1) [4–8].

Early reports of this procedure included photos of patent channels, covered with endothelium [1–3]. However, this theory suffered setbacks as mounting evidence suggested that regardless of the tools used for myocardial puncture (needle, CO_2 laser, Ho:YAG laser), transmyocardial channels did not stay open [9–18]. Thus, most investigators now believe that although patients' symptoms improve, the transmural channels are most often blocked. Mueller *et al.* [19] showed that laser-induced channels were all occluded by a clot at postoperative day 0 and by scar tissue at postoperative day 28, indicating that these channels are obliterated early and do not salvage acute ischemic myocardium. Similarly, Krabatsch *et al.* [20] showed that TMR-created channels were occluded shortly after their creation. Interestingly, the latter study also reported the existence of a developing network of capillaries within areas treated with TMR.

Others have examined the notion that the reduced anginal pain may be because of decreased neural signaling as a result of local denervation. However, despite some evidence suggesting that denervation may be involved [21], a

Table 11.1 Patency rate of TMR channels in various published studies. Summary of most studies in which patency rate of TMR channels is reported. The author, methodology of revascularization, animal model, and author's statement on the patency of observed transmyocardial channels is summarized.

Author [reference]	Method of TMR	Model	Channel patency
Sen, 1965 [2]	Needle	Dogs	Yes
Mirhoseini, 1981 [3]	CO$_2$ laser	Dogs	Yes
Mirhoseini, 1988 [7]	CO$_2$ laser	Humans	Yes
Cooley, 1994 [67]	CO$_2$ laser	Humans	Yes
Horvath, 1995 [68]	CO$_2$ laser	Sheep	Yes
Whittaker, 1996 [69]	Ho:YAG laser + needle	Rats	Yes
Berwing, 1997 [70]	CO$_2$ laser	Humans	Yes
Pifarre, 1969 [69]	Needle	Dogs	No
Owen, 1984 [71]	CO$_2$ laser	Rats	No
Hardy, 1987 [10]	Needle and CO$_2$ laser	Dogs	No
Fleischer, 1996 [11]	CO$_2$ laser	Pigs	No
Kohmoto, 1996 [12]	Ho:YAG laser	Dogs	No
Kohmoto, 1997 [13]	CO$_2$ laser	Dogs	No
Malekan, 1997 [14]	CO$_2$ laser and drill	Sheep	No
Fisher, 1997 [15]	CO$_2$ and Ho:YAG laser	Dogs	No
Yamamoto, 1998 [16]	Ho:YAG laser	Dogs	No
Walpoth, 1998 [17]	CO$_2$, Ho:YAG, erbium laser	Pigs	No
Eckstein, 1998 [18]	Ho:YAG laser	Sheep	No

Ho:YAG, holmium:yttrium-aluminium-garnet.

definitive study by Hirsch *et al.* [22], described in detail elsewhere in this book, showed that TMR does not affect afferent and efferent conductions of cardiac axonal networks, casting doubt on the denervation hypothesis for TMR. Others have supported this view by showing that ST segment changes without chest pain (silent ischemia) did not differ between TMR and medically treated patients during exercise stress testing [23].

The controversies surrounding TMR remain, and to date a consensus on the mechanism(s) has yet to be established. However, neovascularization as the mechanism for reduction of angina by TMR seems to hold considerable support. The rationale is that mechanical injury caused by TMR will initiate the wound healing process with associated angiogenic response and thus improve myocardial tissue perfusion (Fig. 11.1).

The pathophysiology underlying this phenomenon is discussed in some detail below.

Wound healing and angiogenesis

A tissue injury in the body induces a well-defined cascade of events, with the ultimate goal being repair of that tissue. Following the disruption of tissue integrity, either by mechanical injury such as a myocardial puncture, or by hypox-

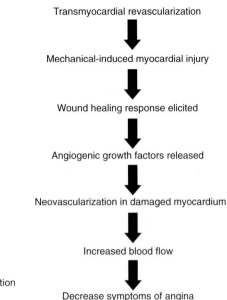

Transmyocardial revascularization

⬇

Mechanical-induced myocardial injury

⬇

Wound healing response elicited

⬇

Angiogenic growth factors released

⬇

Neovascularization in damaged myocardium

⬇

Increased blood flow

⬇

Decrease symptoms of angina

Figure 11.1 Schematic diagram illustrating a hypothesis of the mechanism of angina reduction by transmyocardial revascularization (TMR).

ia as in myocardial infarction, the body responds via activation and proliferation of a subset of cells that aid in the repair and regeneration of native tissue. The mechanisms of such a response, although complex, can be broken into three main components: inflammation, wound remodeling, and angiogenesis.

Inflammatory response to tissue injury

The inflammatory phase of wound healing begins with an initial insult to the tissue. Destruction of capillary endothelium causes transient vasoconstriction of the arterioles followed by vasodilatation. There is increased permeability at the level of the post-capillary venules which allows plasma contents to enter the area of injury [24]. Concurrently, a hemostatic response is activated consisting of both primary and secondary pathways. Primary hemostasis involves platelet aggregation after exposure of the subendothelium and its surface antigen known as von Willebrand factor (VWF), which binds to platelet cell-surface glycoproteins (Gp). Following adhesion of the cells, the platelets undergo a conformational change into pseudopod-like structures where there is rearrangement of the phospholipid membrane and increased expression of GpIIb/IIIa. These glycoprotien moieties allow for binding to fibronectin and platelet aggregation which result in the release of granules containing thromboxane, a potent vasoconstrictor, and other vasoactive factors which activate and attract cells required for wound healing [24]. Thus, platelets provide the initial signals to begin the repair process. Secondary hemostasis involves a delayed clotting cascade initially activated by the exposure of factor VII from the damaged endothelium where it binds to circulating tissue factor [25]. Following a complex cascade of activation of proteins and cleavage of various zymogens, a collection of fibrin monomers are linked to form a thrombus which reinforces the platelet plug formed earlier.

The release of platelet granule contents allow for further reparative processes to occur. Following platelet aggregation, an important cytokine known as platelet-derived growth factor (PDGF) is secreted and serves as the primary chemotactic agent for cells involved in wound healing (polymorphonuclear cells [PMNs], fibroblasts, macrophages, smooth muscle cells), remodeling, and angiogenesis [26,27]. Concomitant changes in vascular permeability combined with changes in Starling forces act synergistically with the endogenous cytokines to cause movement of leukocytes, predominantly PMNs and macrophages, into the underlying interstitium. This process begins with movement towards the walls of the vessels (margination), binding to receptors such as intercellular adhesion molecule 1 (ICAM-1) and selectin protein (adhesion) which causes a conformational change resulting in diapedesis (emigration) into the tissue [28]. Over the next few hours, these cells form an inflammatory exudate within the wound. It is predominantly the macrophages that contribute to further production of cytokines such as interleukins 1–8 (IL-1 to IL-8), endothelial growth factor (EGF), insulin-like growth factor (IGF-1), PDGF, and tumor necrosis factor (TNF) [29]. These cytokines are critical players in further reparative efforts including wound remodeling and the production of new vessels from pre-existing endothelium (i.e., angiogenesis).

Wound remodeling

Wound remodeling occurs as fibroblasts penetrate the damaged area in order to restructure and reconstruct the wounded area. Their migration occurs following activation by cytokines released previously by platelets and macrophages. The fibroblasts secrete glycoproteins and collagen, providing strength to the wound as they are organized into fibers.

Angiogenesis

Following an inflammatory process, many pro-angiogenic proteins are released by the invading platelets and macrophages. Numerous studies have focused on characterizing these angiogenic factors which include cytokines such as IL-2, TNF-a, and growth factors such as vascular endothelial growth factor (VEGF), transforming growth factor b (TGF-b), and basic fibroblast growth factor (bFGF) [30]. Recent progress in understanding the mechanisms of neovascularization indicate that it involves a series of interdependent steps, as discussed below.

Endothelial cells are activated, while concomitant inhibition of apoptosis occurs ensuring their survival for subsequent formation of new vessels. In order to facilitate efficient migration of endothelial cells, many proteases are activated allowing the degradation of the surrounding basement membrane and extracellular matrix. Chemotactic factors that are liberated by platelets, macrophages, neutrophils and fibroblasts allow the endothelial cells to migrate from the proximal parent vessel into areas requiring angiogenesis. Once the endothelial cells have arrived, they proliferate and form tube-like structures and re-differentiate into their original quiescent phenotype. This latter step ensures that the angiogenic process is tightly regulated without formation of superfluous vessels. In order to maintain vessel integrity, the surrounding matrix is reformed under the influence of growth factors such as TGF-b. Now that the angiogenic process is complete, the ischemic area can receive increased blood flow via the newly formed vascular conduit.

Overview of vascular growth factors

For over three decades, a variety of proteins have been identified that cause the formation of new vascular structures. These growth factors include three main families of peptides: fibroblast growth factors (FGF), vascular endothelial growth factors (VEGF) and, more recently, the angiopoetins.

Fibroblast growth factors

The FGF family of angiogenic mediators consists of over twenty different proteins, each sharing sequence and structural homogeneity. They are characterized by high-affinity binding to both heparin and cells expressing tyrosine kinase activity [31]. They have important roles in angiogenesis, mitogenesis, cellular differentiation, and wound healing. Only FGF-1 (acidic FGF/aFGF) and FGF-2 (basic FGF/bFGF) are expressed at high levels in adults. FGF-1 expression is predominantly confined to the central nervous system, but FGF-2 is ubiquitously expressed throughout all adult tissues [32].

The cellular mechanisms responsible for their angiogenic action have also been well documented. Upon binding to the specific FGF receptors, they initiate a variety of cascades that result in activation of proteases essential for matrix degradation, inhibition of endothelial apoptosis, and kinase activation responsible for cell replication and secretion of signaling molecules involved in tubule formation [33]. Recent studies have shown that TMR-treated myocardium demonstrates increased expression of bFGF in mice along with increased formation of new blood vessels [34]. Others have shown that the ability of TMR to promote angiogenesis in damaged myocardium is increased following concomitant treatment with bFGF [35].

Vascular endothelial growth factors

In 1989, two separate laboratories identified an endothelial cell-specific mitogen which they called vascular endothelial growth factor (VEGF), formerly known as vasculotropin or vascular permeability factor (VPF) [36,37]. Currently, six splice variants of VEGF have been identified in which they share common motifs and a dimeric glycoprotein quaternary structure [38]. However, these isoforms differ with respect to their chemotactic properties, growth factor interactions, heparin binding, and mitogenicity. Primarily, these proteins have two major effects on endothelial cellular mechanics. Of paramount importance to our discussion is their ability to induce endothelial cell proliferation. Stimulation of endothelial cells with VEGF allows the production of a new subset of cells for the formation of new vessels [39]. Furthermore, the growth factor also demonstrates a strong chemotactic ability to guide endothelial cells to areas requiring angiogenesis [40].

VEGF expression is partly regulated by O_2 tension, which provides a regulatory feedback mechanism for blood vessel formation. This process of hypoxic-induced VEGF expression is of much interest in current literature, and appears to be regulated by a group of genes called hypoxia inducible factors (HIF) [41]. These HIF peptides bind to response elements in the VEGF promoter which up-regulate VEGF expression during times of low O_2 tension.

Angiopoetins

It was only recently that a new group of biologic mediators were identified as having angiogenic properties. This family of four proteins share common coil-coiled and fibrinogen-like domains, and bind to the endothelial receptor tyrosine kinase Tie2 [42]. However, their effects after binding Tie2 are different for the various isoforms. Two of these proteins, angiopoetin 1 and 4 (Ang-1, Ang-4), activate the receptor whereas Ang-2 and Ang-3 inhibit Tie2 activation [31]. These opposing actions are thought to add another element to the regulation of the angiogenic process. Functional disruption of the angiopoietin receptor results in embryonic lethality at E10 and illustrates the importance of Tie2 in angiogenesis and hematopoiesis in early development [43].

Interestingly, Ang-2 but not Ang-1 expression is upregulated during times of low O_2 tension. Furthermore, these proteins are also differentially regulated by other angiogenic growth factors such as bFGF and VEGF [44,45]. Similar to hypoxic-induced angiopoietin expression, these growth factors have been shown to increase Ang-2 expression without effecting Ang-1 levels. Although many questions remain unanswered, recent research indicates that this family of proteins have important roles in the maturation of new blood vessels formed by angiogenesis.

Angiogenesis in TMR

The idea of angiogenesis as a sequel to the injury caused by TMR has gained considerable interest and subsequently has been the focus of intense research efforts. Despite this, much uncertainty remains regarding whether any observed increase in histologic revascularization is associated with an increase in perfusion. At the root of the "pro-angiogenesis argument" as the main mechanism of TMR, clear proof of increased perfusion must be demonstrated. While there are good animal data to support this, the same cannot be said of human trials. Nonetheless, there is substantial evidence that TMR-induced angiogenesis results from the increased expression of vascular growth factors, in itself a non-specific inflammatory response to myocardial injury.

Evidence of angiogenesis by histology

Histologic and hemodynamic studies in animals have illustrated that TMR enhances angiogenesis above that normally seen in ischemic myocardium. Chu *et al.* [46] demonstrated that VEGF expression and new vessel formation were increased in pigs following chronic constriction of the circumflex artery and concomitant treatment with TMR using a 25-gauge needle. Furthermore, histologic evidence demonstrated that virtually none of the channels remained patent. In further studies by this group, Pelletier *et al.* [47] also showed that bFGF and TGF-b expression was upregulated following similar treatment. Besides vascular growth factors, studies have shown that other mediators in the angiogenic response are also activated following TMR. The role of nitric oxide (NO) in the wound repair as a promoter of endothelial cell proliferation and migration has been well documented [48]. Saito *et al.* [49] investigated the expression profiles of both inducible and endothelial nitric oxide synthetases (iNOS and eNOS, respectively) following needle-induced TMR. After ligation of the LAD, they showed that rats treated concomitantly with TMR had higher expression of iNOS, higher macrophage infiltration, and higher levels of vascular density. This study illustrated that iNOS may be an important mediator in the angiogenic process following TMR while also correlating the response to the inflammatory process.

Similar studies have been carried out in higher animal models, with the ultimate goal of creating a therapeutic regimen optimal for use in humans. Malekan *et al.* [50], examined the possibility that angiogenesis also occurs in ovine myocardium following TMR-induced injury. In this experiment, sheep underwent creation of transmyocardial channels in the left ventricle through the use of both CO_2 laser and a power drill in the alternate region of the same heart. All original transmural channels were closed at 4 weeks. Histologic examination showed channel remnants composed of fibrosis, granulation tissue, and new capillary formation, and these changes were similar for both methods of channel creation. New smooth muscle media was observed and densities of the vessels within the channel remnants were both significantly greater than the density of vessels in remote regions. Another study was performed on an explanted human heart 6 months after TMR therapy. The investigators examined histologic sections and identified newly formed vessels in the channel remnant and adjacent to the sites of injury [51]. Immunohistochemical staining verified the presence of endothelial cell markers and erythrocytes were visualized within these newly formed vessels. This was one of the longest TMR follow-up investigations showing the pro-angiogenic effects of the procedure.

Together, these studies have provided strong evidence that new blood vessel formation occurs following injury produced by TMR. The release of angiogenic growth factors appears to mediate this process. But does this leads to improved tissue perfusion?

Evidence of angiogenesis by tissue perfusion studies

To embrace angiogenesis as the leading mechanism of TMR, proof of increased perfusion must be demonstrated. It is not adequate to demonstrate increased levels of angiogenic growth factors or increased vascular density. There are several studies demonstrating a significant improvement in perfusion in animals, mostly in pigs (Table 11.2).

In the acute phase, Lutter *et al*. [52] in 1998 were unable to demonstrate an increase in perfusion. Pigs were treated with TMR (CO_2, 40 J) prior to occlusion of the LAD, and perfusion was studied with microspheres. Compared with a control group, there was no increase in regional myocardial blood flow, despite fewer ventricular arrhythmias and less myocardial necrosis. However, in a separate chronic experiment, the same group demonstrated an increase in tissue perfusion [53]. After inducing a stenosis in the LAD, pigs were treated with CO_2 TMR and perfusion was measured by radioactive microsperes. After 3 months, regional myocardial blood flow was significantly higher in the TMR group compared with the ischemia control group (0.39 ± 0.13 vs 0.14 ± 0.12 mL/min/g; $P = 0.043$).

A study by Hamawy *et al*. [54] used ^{99m}Tc-sestamibi scans to demonstrate increased perfusion in a chronic myocardial ischemia model. Twelve swine underwent placement of an ameroid constrictor around the circumflex artery to create a localized area of ischemia. The animals then underwent a TMR procedure through a thoracotomy, followed by sestamibi perfusion scans 4 weeks later. Semi-quantitative analyses of the perfusion scan demonstrate significant improvement ($P < 0.04$) in stress-induced ischemia in animals with 50 TMR channels, but not in animals with either 25 or 10 channels. In the 50-channel group, a $42 \pm 22\%$ improvement in the area of ischemia was noted. The authors concluded that myocardial perfusion was enhanced in this animal model, and suggested that a dose–response relationship related to channel number may be of significance.

Table 11.2 Summary of perfusion studies for transmyocardial revascularization.

Model	Laser	Timing	Method	Perfusion improvement	Reference
Swine	Excimer	4 weeks	SPECT	Yes	54
Porcine	Excimer	12 weeks	Radioactive microspheres	Yes	55
Porcine	CO_2	6 months	PET	Yes	56
Porcine	CO_2	8 weeks	MRI	Yes	57
Rats	CO_2	12 weeks	MRI	Yes	58
Porcine	CO_2	3 months	Radioactive microspheres	Yes	53
Humans	CO_2	3, 6 months	SPECT	Yes	59
Human	CO_2	3, 12 months	SPECT	No	61
Human	CO_2	6, 12 months	SPECT	No	62
Human	CO_2	7, 34 weeks	PET	No	63
Porcine	CO_2	12 weeks	Microspheres	No	61

CO_2, carbon dioxide laser; MRI, magnetic resonance imaging; PET, positron emission tomography; SPECT, technetium-99m tetrofosmin myocardial perfusion tomography.

In a similar porcine model of chronic ischemia, Martin *et al.* [55] compared the efficacy of CO_2 and excimer lasers by measuring regional myocardial blood flow (RMBF) with radioactive microspheres 12 weeks after treatment. In the ischemic zone, RMBF (mL/min/g) was improved in both the CO_2 (0.73 ± 0.19) and excimer (0.78 ± 0.22) groups when compared with controls (0.55 ± 0.12; $P < 0.05$).

By using positron emission tomography (PET), a group from Duke University was also able to demonstrate increased perfusion [56]. Using a miniswine model with subtotal occlusion of the circumflex artery, animals underwent TMR 2 weeks after creating the ischemic event. PET scanning demonstrated a significant improvement in myocardial blood flow to the lased region 6 months postoperatively.

With yet another method to assess perfusion, Muhling *et al.* [57] studied myocardial perfusion in pigs using quantitative magnetic resonance perfusion imaging (MRPI). Twelve pigs underwent partial occlusion of the circumflex artery and subsequently randomized to either TMR or control groups. The animals were studied 8 weeks later with MRPI. Resting perfusion prior to TMLR (0.7–0.9 ± 0.3) in the left ventricular lateral myocardium was preserved after TMLR (1.0 ± 0.3) and decreased without TMLR (0.3 ± 0.1; $P < 0.05$). The authors concluded that TMLR preserves regional myocardial perfusion and improves function as shown with MRPI.

Nahrendorf *et al.* [58] have used a rat ischemia model and MRPI to demonstrate a significant perfusion improvement after TMLR. Eight weeks after ligation of the coronary artery, TMLR was performed in the remote myocardium. Twelve weeks later, MRPI was performed at rest and during nitroglycerin-induced stress in the TMLR group. TMLR-treated areas were better perfused than untreated myocardium (3.89 ± 0.83 mL/min/g at rest vs. 2.29 ± 1.06 mL/min/g; $P < 0.05$) during nitroglycerin-induced stress.

In humans, a study of 15 patients who underwent TMLR and ^{99m}Tc-MIBI scintigraphy revealed improved perfusion of 33.7% of the transient defects within 3 months after TMLR, which persisted at 6 months with a clear trend towards further improvement in the lased segments [59].

Despite all of these studies suggesting that perfusion is improved, other studies have contradicted these findings. Lutter *et al.* [60] demonstrated an improvement in regional myocardial blood flow 12 weeks after TMLR in a chronic pig ischemia model. However, no absolute improvement in perfusion at rest compared with baseline was observed in these experimental groups.

For proponents of the improved perfusion, the main obstacle has been to demonstrate this objectively in humans, where findings of improved perfusion have yet to be clearly demonstrated. A study performed in Norway randomized 100 patients with refractory angina to either TMR (CO_2 laser) or medical therapy [61]. By using technetium-99m tetrofosmin myocardial perfusion tomography (SPECT) scans, no significant difference in perfusion could be found between groups after 3 and 12 months. In fact, the authors found a slight reduction in left ventricular ejection fraction and an increase in left ventricular end-diastolic volume in the TMR group. Similar results were noted by Lutter *et al.* [62] in a report of 62 patients who underwent either TMLR + CABG or TMLR alone. Radionuclide assessment failed to demonstrate any difference in perfusion in the lasered ischemic segments at 6 and 12 months.

Yet another study in humans has failed to demonstrate improved myocardial perfusion [63]. Myocardial blood flow (MBF) was measured by means of PET in seven patients with refractory angina before and after CO_2 TMLR. Resting MBF (MBFR) in both lasered and non-lasered regions was unchanged after TMLR. Despite an improvement in anginal symptoms, MBF was not seen to be higher at 7.5 and 34.6 weeks postoperatively.

In summarizing the available data, there is a general consensus that long-term improvements in myocardial perfusion have yet to be demonstrated in humans [60–63], despite some very good animal data to suggest otherwise [53–58]. Either there is some improvement in perfusion and the wrong methodology has been used, or there is truly no change in long-term perfusion. For now, one must consider the prospect of angiogenesis as a possibility that has yet to be conclusively proven.

Future studies

In order to clearly demonstrate the long-term angiogenic potential of TMR, a proper randomized trial must be undertaken aimed at assessing perfusion. Using nuclear imaging, angiography, or MRI studies, it must be demonstrated that TMR-treated myocardium exhibits increased perfusion to these areas over the long term. As studies progress to develop the ultimate modality for delivering TMR to injured myocardium, there should also be parallel studies to show which modality of punctures will display the maximum angiogenic response. For example, few studies have compared the long-term angiogenic response in CO_2 laser verses holmium:yttrium-aluminium-garnet laser or needle-delivered TMR [47,64,65]. In such comparative studies, the dose–response relationship, and the magnitude of angiogenesis versus tissue damage, the latter potentially harmful, should be taken into consideration. Some have also suggested the potential for TMR therapy with concomitant pro-angiogenic cytokine therapy with the hopes of a synergistic effect to increase TMR efficacy [66]. Thus, the refinement of an appropriate delivery system and angiogenic cytokine therapy would be an important step to provide patients with the most effective care.

As the field of myocardial revascularization expands and the number of patients not amenable to current techniques increases, the addition of TMR to our therapeutic armamentarium will potentially become increasingly popular. It is important to decipher the mechanism by which TMR can improve symptoms of ischemic heart disease so that we can maximize the efficacy of this novel approach.

References

1 Sen PK, Daulatram J, Kinare SG, Udwadia TE, Parulkar GB. Further studies in multiple transmyocardial acupuncture as a method of myocardial revascularization. *Surgery* 1968;**64**:861–70.

2 Sen PK, Udwadia TE, Kinare SG, Parulkar GB. Transmyocardial acupuncture: a new approach to myocardial revascularization. *J Thorac Cardiovasc Surg* 1965;**50**:181–9.

3 Mirhoseini M, Cayton M. Revascularization of the heart by laser. *J Microsurg* 1981;**2**: 871–5.

4 Mirhoseini M, Muckerheide M, Cayton M. Transventricular revascularization by laser. *Lasers Surg Med* 1982;**2**:187–98.

5 Mirhoseini M, Fisher JC, Cayton M. Myocardial revascularization by laser: a clinical report. *Lasers Surg Med* 1983;**3**:241–5.

6 Mirhoseini M, Cayton M, Shelgikar S, Fisher JC. Clinical report: laser myocardial revascularization. *Lasers Surg Med* 1986;**6**:459–61.

7 Mihroseini M, Shelgikar S, Cayton M. New concepts in revascularization of the myocardium. *Ann Thorac Surg* 1988;**4**:415–20.

8 Mirhoseini M, Shelgikar S, Cayton M. Clinical and histological evaluation of laser myocardial revascularization. *J Clin Laser Med Surg* 1990;**6**:73–8.

9 Pifarre R, Jasuja ML, Lynch RD, Neville WE. Myocardial revascularization by transmyocardial acupuncture: a physiologic impossibility. *J Thorac Cardiovasc Surg* 1969;**58**:424–31.

10 Hardy RI, Bove KE, James FW, Kaplan S, Goldman L. A histologic study of laser-induced transmyocardial channels. *Lasers Surg Med* 1987;**6**:563–73.

11 Fleischer K, Goldschmidt-Clermont PJ, Fonger JG, *et al.* One-month histologic response of transmyocardial laser channels with molecular intervention. *Ann Thorac Surg* 1996;**62**: 1051–8.

12 Kohmoto T, Fisher PE, Gu A, *et al.* Does blood flow through Holmium:YAG transmyocardial laser channels? *Ann Thorac Surg* 1996;**61**:861–8.

13 Kohmoto T, Fisher PE, Gu A, *et al.* Physiology, histology, and 2-week morphology of acute transmyocardial channels made with a CO_2 laser. *Ann Thorac Surg* 1997;**63**:1275–83.

14 Malekan R, Reynolds C, Kelley S, *et al.* Angiogenesis in transmyocardial laser revascularization: a nonspecific response to injury. *Circulation* 1997;**96**(Suppl 1):564.

15 Fisher P, Khomoto T, DeRosa C, *et al.* Histologic analysis of transmyocardial channels: comparison of CO2 and Holmium:YAG lasers. *Ann Thorac Surg* 1997;**64**:466–72.

16 Yamamoto N, Kohmoto T, Gu A, *et al.* Angigenesis is enhanced in ischemic canine myocardium by transmyocardial laser revascularization. *J Am Coll Cardiol* 1998;**31**:1426–33.

17 Walpoth BH, Genyk I, Aeschbacher B, *et al.* Comparison of 3 different laser techniques for transmyocardial revascularization in the pig (Abstract). Presented at the 12th Annual Meeting of the European Association for Cardio-thoracic Surgery, Brussels, Belgium, 1998.

18 Eckstein F, Scheule A, Vogel U, *et al.* Transmyocardial laser revascularization with the Homium:YAG laser in the acute ischemic heart does neither improve acute myocardial perfusion nor does it prevent from myocardial infarction. An experimental study. Presented at the 12th Annual Meeting of the European Association for Cardio-thoracic Surgery, Brussels, Belgium, 1998.

19 Mueller XM, Tevaearai HT, Chaubert P, Genton CY, von Segesser LK. [Mechanism of action of transmyocardial laser revascularization (animal experiment)]. *Schweiz Med Wochenschr* 1999;**129**:1889–92.

20 Krabatsch T, Schaper F, Leder C, *et al.* Histological findings after transmyocardial laser revascularization. *J Card Surg* 1996;**11**:326–31.

21 Kwong KF, Kanellopoulos GK, Nickols JC, *et al.* Transmyocardial laser treatment denervates canine myocardium. *J Thorac Cardiovasc Surg* 1997;**114**:883–9.

22 Hirsch GM, Thompson GW, Arora RC, *et al.* Transmyocardial laser revascularization does not denervate the canine heart. *Ann Thorac Surg* 1999;**68**:460–8.

23 Myers J, Oesterle SN, Jones J, Burkhoff D. Do transmyocardial and percutaneous laser revascularization induce silent ischemia? An assessment by exercise testing. *Am Heart J* 2002;**143**:1052–7.

24 Troy GC. An overview of hemostasis. *Vet Clin North Am Small Anim Pract* 1988;**18**:5–20.

25 Rusconi CP, Yeh A, Lyerly HK, Lawson JH, Sullenger BA. Blocking the initiation of coagulation by RNA aptamers to factor VIIa. *Thromb Haemost* 2000;**84**:841–8.

26 Heldin CH, Westermark B. Mechanism of action and *in vivo* role of platelet-derived growth factor. *Physiol Rev* 1999;**79**:1283–316.

27 Pierce GF, Mustoe TA, Altrock BW, Deuel TF, Thomason A. Role of platelet-derived growth factor in wound healing. *J Cell Biochem* 1991;**45**:319–26.

28 Subramaniam M, Saffaripour S, Van De WL, *et al.* Role of endothelial selectins in wound repair. *Am J Pathol* 1997;**150**:1701–9.

29 Gillitzer R, Goebeler M. Chemokines in cutaneous wound healing. *J Leukoc Biol* 2001;**69**:513–21.

30 Bernardini G, Ribatti D, Spinetti G, *et al.* Analysis of the role of chemokines in angiogenesis. *J Immunol Methods* 2003;**273**:83–101.

31 Kutryk MJB SD. Pharmacologic revascularization. In: Theroux P (ed.) *Brunwald's Companion Textbook on Acute Coronary Syndromes*. Philadelphia: W.B.Saunders Company, 2003.

32 Szebenyi G, Fallon JF. Fibroblast growth factors as multifunctional signaling factors. *Int Rev Cytol* 1999;**185**:45–106.

33 Nugent MA, Iozzo RV. Fibroblast growth factor-2. *Int J Biochem Cell Biol* 2000;**32**:115–20.

34 Chiotti K, Choo SJ, Martin SL, *et al.* Activation of myocardial angiogenesis and upregulation of fibroblast growth factor-2 in transmyocardial-revascularization-treated mice. *Coron Artery Dis* 2000;**11**:537–44.

35 Yamamoto N, Kohmoto T, Roethy W, *et al.* Histologic evidence that basic fibroblast growth factor enhances the angiogenic effects of transmyocardial laser revascularization. *Basic Res Cardiol* 2000;**95**:55–63.

36 Ferrara N, Henzel WJ. Pituitary follicular cells secrete a novel heparin-binding growth factor specific for vascular endothelial cells. *Biochem Biophys Res Commun* 1989;**161**: 851–8.

37 Plouet J, Schilling J, Gospodarowicz D. Isolation and characterization of a newly identified endothelial cell mitogen produced by AtT-20 cells. *EMBO J* 1989;**8**:3801–6.

38 Stimpfl M, Tong D, Fasching B, *et al.* Vascular endothelial growth factor splice variants and their prognostic value in breast and ovarian cancer. *Clin Cancer Res* 2002;**8**:2253–9.

39 Buschmann I, Heil M, Jost M, Schaper W. Influence of inflammatory cytokines on arteriogenesis. *Microcirculation* 2003;**10**:371–9.

40 Asahara T, Takahashi T, Masuda H, *et al.* VEGF contributes to postnatal neovascularization by mobilizing bone marrow-derived endothelial progenitor cells. *EMBO J* 1999;**18**:3964–72.

41 Semenza GL. Regulation of hypoxia-induced angiogenesis: a chaperone escorts VEGF to the dance. *J Clin Invest* 2001;**108**:39–40.

42 Davis S, Yancopoulos GD. The angiopoietins: Yin and Yang in angiogenesis. *Curr Top Microbiol Immunol* 1999;**237**:173–85.

43 Puri MC, Partanen J, Rossant J, Bernstein A. Interaction of the TEK and TIE receptor tyrosine kinases during cardiovascular development. *Development* 1999;**126**:4569–80.

44 Enholm B, Paavonen K, Ristimaki A, *et al*. Comparison of VEGF, VEGF-B, VEGF-C and Ang-1 mRNA regulation by serum, growth factors, oncoproteins and hypoxia. *Oncogene* 1997;**14**:2475–83.

45 Tsigkos S, Koutsilieris M, Papapetropoulos A. Angiopoietins in angiogenesis and beyond. *Expert Opin Investig Drugs* 2003;**12**:933–41.

46 Chu VF, Giaid A, Kuang JQ, *et al*. Thoracic Surgery Directors Association Award. Angiogenesis in transmyocardial revascularization: comparison of laser versus mechanical punctures. *Ann Thorac Surg* 1999;**68**:301–7.

47 Pelletier MP, Giaid A, Sivaraman S, *et al*. Angiogenesis and growth factor expression in a model of transmyocardial revascularization. *Ann Thorac Surg* 1998;**66**:12–8.

48 Schwentker A, Billiar TR. Nitric oxide and wound repair. *Surg Clin North Am* 2003;**83**:521–30.

49 Saito T, Pelletier MP, Shennib H, Giaid A. Nitric oxide system in needle-induced transmyocardial revascularization. *Ann Thorac Surg* 2001;**72**:129–36.

50 Malekan R, Reynolds C, Narula N, *et al*. Angiogenesis in transmyocardial laser revascularization. A nonspecific response to injury. *Circulation* 1998;**98**(Suppl 2):62–5.

51 Domkowski PW, Biswas SS, Steenbergen C, Lowe JE. Histological evidence of angiogenesis 9 months after transmyocardial laser revascularization. *Circulation* 2001;**103**:469–71.

52 Lutter G, Yoshitake M, Takahashi N, *et al*. Transmyocardial laser-revascularization: experimental studies on prolonged acute regional ischemia. *Eur J Cardiothorac Surg* 1998;**13**; 694–701.

53 Lutter G, Martin J, von Samson P, *et al*. Microperfusion enhancement after TMLR in chronically ischemic porcine hearts. *Cardiovasc Surg* 2001;**9**:281–91.

54 Hamawy AH, Lee LY, Samy SA, *et al*. Transmyocardial laser revascularization dose response: enhanced perfusion in a porcine ischemia model as a function of channel density. *Ann Thorac Surg* 2001;**72**:817–22.

55 Martin JS, Sayeed-Shah U, Byrne JG, *et al*. Excimer versus carbon dioxide transmyocardial laser revascularization: effects on regional left ventricular function and perfusion. *Ann Thorac Surg* 2000;**69**:1811–6.

56 Hughes GC, Kypson AP, St. Louis JD, *et al*. Improved perfusion and contractile reserve after transmyocardial laser revascularization in a model of hibernating myocardium. *Ann Thorac Surg* 2000;**67**:1714–20.

57 Muhling OM, Wang Y, Panse P, *et al*. Transmyocardial laser revascularization preserves regional myocardial perfusion: an MRI first pass perfusion study. *Cardiovasc Res* 2003;**57**: 63–70.

58 Nahrendorf M, Hiller KH, Theisen D, *et al*. Effect of transmyocardial laser revascularization on myocardial perfusion and left ventricular remodeling after myocardial infarction in rats. *Radiology* 2002;**225**:487–93.

59 Kostkiewicz M, Rudzinski P, Tracz W, Dziatkowiak A. Changes in myocardial perfuison after transmyocardial laser revascularization in patients with end-stage angina pectoris. *Cardiology* 2000;**94**:173–8.

60 Lutter G, Martin J, Dern P, *et al*. Evaluation of the indirect revascularization method after 3 months chronic myocardial ischemia. *Eur J Cardiothorac Surg* 2000;**18**:38–45.

61 Aaberge L, Rootwelt K, Smith HJ, Nordstrand K, Forfang K. Effects of transmyocardial revascularization on myocardial perfusion and systolic function assessed by nuclear and magnetic resonance imaging methods. *Scand Cardiovasc J* 2001;**35**:8–13.

62 Lutter G, Sarai K, Nitzsche E, *et al*. Evaluation of transmyocardial laser revascularization by following objective parameters of perfusion and ventricular function. *Thorac Cardiovasc Surg* 2000;**48**:79–85.

63 Rimoldi O, Burns SM, Rosen SD, *et al*. Measurement of myocardial blood flow with positron emission tomography before and after transmyocardial laser revascularization. *Circulation* 1999;**100**:II134–8.

64 Hughes GC, Biswas SS, Yin B, *et al*. A comparison of mechanical and laser transmyocardial revascularization for induction of angiogenesis and arteriogenesis in chronically ischemic myocardium. *J Am Coll Cardiol* 2002;**39**:1220–8.

65 Hughes GC, Kypson AP, Annex BH, *et al*. Induction of angiogenesis after TMR: a comparison of holmium: YAG, CO2, and excimer lasers. *Ann Thorac Surg* 2000;**70**:504–9.

66 Horvath KA, Doukas J, Belkind N, *et al*. Restoration of myocardial function with combination angiogenesis therapy. *Heart Surg Forum* 2003;**6**(Suppl 1):S39.

67 Cooley DA, Frazier OH, Kadipasaoglu KA, *et al*. Transmyocardial laser revascularization: anatomic evidence of long-term channel patency. *Tex Heart Inst J* 1994;**21**:220–4.

68 Horvath KA, Smith WJ, Laurence RG, *et al*. Recovery and viability of an acute myocardial infarct after transmyocardial laser revascularization. *J Am Coll Cardiol* 1995;**25**:258–63.

69 Whittaker P, Rakusan K, Kloner RA. Transmural channels can protect ischemic tissue: Assessment of long-term myocardial response to laser- and needle-made channels. *Circulation* 1996;**93**:143–52.

70 Berwing K, Bauer E, Strasser R, *et al*. Functional evidence of long-term channel patency after transmyocardial laser revascularization. *Circulation* 1997;**96**:I-564.

71 Owen ER, Canfield P, Bryant K, Hopwood PR. Observations on the effects of CO2-laser on rat myocardium. *Microsurgery* 1984;**5**:140–3.

CHAPTER 12

Myocardial sinusoids and non-compaction: embryology and relevance to the adult coronary circulation

Ray CJ Chiu, Stephen J Korkola, and Kevin Lachapelle

Introduction

For over half a century, the nature of the vascular communications in the heart described by Wearn *et al.* [1] in the 1930s has been cited as the basis for a number of surgical interventions for myocardial revascularization. The purpose of this review is to demonstrate those conditions in which persistent myocardial sinusoids clearly exist, and can be diagnosed today, in definable pathologic hearts. We review phylogenetic and embryonal developments, and describe certain congenital anomalies of the coronary circulation where vascular communications exist between the coronary circulation and the ventricular lumen, and discuss their clinical relevance.

Myocardial sinusoids in the human heart

Development of the sinusoidal concept

Wearn *et al.* [1] studied human hearts at autopsy by the injection of colored gelatins and celloidan at supernormal pressures in the ventricular chambers and coronary arteries. They described a number of vascular communications in the heart in meticulous detail. These communications were thought to represent an interconnecting network between the coronary arteries, the ventricular chamber, and the myocardial "sinusoids." The intimate association of sinusoids with the muscle fibers was thought to be evidence of their importance in normal myocardial oxygenation.

Treating ischemic heart disease with myocardial sinusoids

The Vineberg procedure

The Vineberg procedure was one of the early surgical treatments proposed for coronary artery disease [2]. It was based on the presence of the myocardial sinusoidal network described by Wearn. Vineberg relied on this concept when he implanted the internal mammary artery (IMA) directly into the ischemic myocardium. He believed that the implanted IMA graft would remain patent because of the pre-existing distal run-off provided by the sponge-like myocardium with prevalent sinusoids [3]. Other investigators [4] implanted plastic T-tubes into the myocardium to conduct ventricular blood into the sinusoids for the purpose of myocardial revascularization.

Transmyocardial revascularization
Another surgical procedure based on the sinusoidal concept in the heart has been revived recently with the popularization of transmyocardial revascularization (TMR). Sen *et al.* [5] originally attempted TMR in the 1960s by performing transmyocardial acupuncture with a needle, trying to recreate the reptilian myocardial vascular pattern. Thus, this procedure was nicknamed the "snake heart operation." The snake myocardium is supplied from the ventricular cavity during systole as blood is forced from the ventricle into a rich sinusoidal network that bathes the cardiomyocytes. Sen tried to recreate this pattern of myocardial perfusion by creating transmural channels in ischemic myocardium with a needle, attempting to perfuse the heart with blood flowing through the channels from the ventricular cavity and into the myocardial sinusoids. He obtained promising results in the acutely ischemic dog model, reporting smaller infarcts and better survival in the TMR group. However, after Sen's initial work, others had difficulty showing that channels created with a needle would remain patent over time [6], a prerequisite for the procedure's success if the snake-heart concept was indeed valid. The enthusiasm over needle TMR faded for a period because of concerns with lack of channel patency and because other methods of direct revascularization were being developed [7,8]. However, there was a resurgence in the concept of TMR during the 1980s when Mirhoseini and Cayton [9] proposed that the CO_2 laser had special properties that would make it useful for creating transmural channels in the myocardium. The reasoning behind how laser TMR should work was that these channels, created by certain laser energy, unlike needle punctures, would remain open to perfuse the myocardial sinusoidal network. They demonstrated favorable results in animal models [9] and later in human studies where they combined laser TMR with coronary artery bypass grafting (CABG) [10]. Industry seized the opportunity afforded by the findings in early studies and began to develop laser equipment specifically designed to create TMR channels. Over the last 10 years considerable investment of time and money has been devoted to developing TMR, and several clinical trials have been carried out, some with favorable results, yet there is little evidence for the existence of myocardial sinusoids in humans [11] except in exceptional circumstances [12–14]. Increasingly, however, the idea of TMR working through patent channels perfusing the myocardium directly is coming into doubt [15,16].

Evolution of the myocardial blood supply

Myocardial vascular patterns

Observations made in a number of animal species have revealed wide variation in myocardial vascular patterns depending on the evolutionary stage of the animal. From cold-blooded reptiles to warm-blooded vertebrates, there is a spectrum of vascular patterns that can be generally classified into four types in an ascending order of complexity [17].

The first type has been termed a *sinusoidal type* in which all of the myocardial perfusion comes directly from the ventricular chamber. Blood is forced from the ventricular chamber into a spongy sinusoidal network that is intimately associated with the myocardial cells. This sinusoidal network is a collection of endothelial-lined spaces that are perfused with ventricular blood during systole. This blood is recirculated back into the ventricle during diastole, as there are no other developed conduits to serve as the outflow for this blood.

The second vascular pattern has been termed *transitional type I* in which the outer layer of myocardium has become compacted and is supplied by coronary arteries, a well-developed capillary bed, and coronary veins. This outer compact layer coexists with an inner layer of spongy myocardium which is supplied from the ventricular blood and sinusoids in the manner described above.

The third myocardial vascular pattern is called *transitional type II*, with an outer compact layer of muscle supplied by the coronary arteries and an inner non-compacted layer that is supplied both from the ventricular and sinusoidal network as well as from branches of the coronary arteries penetrating the trabeculations.

The final type is a *coronary type* in which the entire myocardium has undergone compaction and is supplied from a well-developed coronary artery–capillary network.

The first three patterns are found in cold-blooded animals while the more efficient coronary type has evolved in warm-blooded vertebrates to cope with higher metabolic demands [17]. During development of the mammalian fetus, it has been observed that the heart progresses through the above stages to end with a mature coronary circulation and no residual sinusoidal circulation [18].

Embryology of mammalian myocardial vascular system

The development of the vascular patterns in the mammalian heart has been well described in a widely quoted article by Grant [18]. In the early embryonal development of the heart, the myocardium is formed as a spongy trabecular network supplied with blood from the ventricular chamber perfusing abundant myocardial sinusoids. The spongy myocardium then begins to undergo "compaction." The coronary veins develop first and establish communications with the deep intertrabecular recesses and sinusoidal network. The coronary arteries follow, establishing connections with the aorta, sinusoids, and veins. This is occurring as the myocardium is undergoing compaction to obliterate sinusoids in an orderly and predictable sequence. Compaction proceeds from base to apex, from posterior to anterior, from right to left ventricle, and from epicardium to endocardium [19]. Thus, the left ventricular apex is the last area of the heart to assume the mature compact ventricular myocardium seen in the adult heart. It should also be noted that while the compaction process begins in the right ventricle, it is less complete there and some trabeculations persist in the normal adult right ventricle [20]. The development of the human heart can be viewed as a time line of the evolutionary process. In the early developmental stages, it resembles the primitive heart of reptiles (the "snake heart") but increases in complexity and efficiency to become the compacted mammalian heart supplied by the well-developed coronary arterial system.

Persistence of primitive vascular patterns in the human

Primitive myocardial perfusion patterns have repeatedly been cited in the surgical literature as targets for revascularizing ischemic myocardium. These patterns do persist in the form of abnormal communications of the coronary arteries with the ventricular chambers, persistence of myocardial sinusoids, and failure of the ventricular myocardium to undergo compaction. However, these conditions are extremely rare and are associated with undesirable consequences rather than beneficial effects.

Coronary artery–ventricular fistulae

A 70-year-old woman with no history of cardiac disease presented to the hospital with new-onset retrosternal chest pain, radiating to the jaw, which awoke her from sleep. Electrocardiography (ECG) showed sinus rhythm with a few premature ventricular beats and no evidence of ischemic changes. All blood work, including serial cardiac enzymes, was within normal limits. The pain lasted 12 hours, being relieved eventually with intravenous morphine. Selective coronary arteriogram revealed numerous coronary–left ventricular cavity fistulae, originating from a large first obtuse marginal branch of the circumflex coronary artery (Fig. 12.1a) as well as from the distal posterior ventricular branch of the right coronary artery (Fig. 12.1b). There were no significant stenoses of any coronary arteries. A transthoracic echocardiogram revealed normal ventricular dimensions, wall thickness, and systolic function with an ejection fraction of 60%. There were no valvular abnormalities demonstrated. She was started on acetylsalicylic acid and β-blockers and has remained asymptomatic since.

The above case report illustrates the persistence of direct communications of the coronary arteries with the ventricular chamber. Although such communications, which can be demonstrated by angiography today, were described in the adult human heart by Wearn's classic study [1], they are rare and their significance has not been determined. The developing coronary arteries establish communication with the trabecular sinusoidal network in the fetal heart. It has been suggested that developmental arrest in localized areas of myocardium leads to persistence of such communications [21]. There have been a number of case reports of these communications persisting as an isolated condition

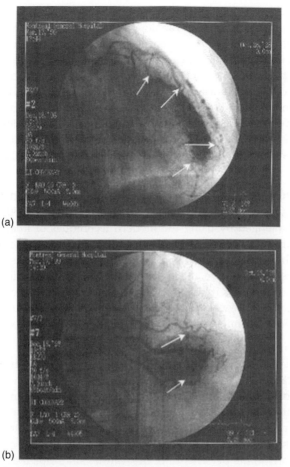

Figure 12.1 (a) Right anterior oblique (RAO) projection of left coronary arteriogram demonstrating multiple small fistulae between the circumflex coronary artery and the left ventricular chamber. (b) Left anterior oblique (LAO) projection of right coronary artery injection revealing fistulous communications between the posterior ventricular branch of the right coronary artery and the left ventricular chamber.

[22–29]. The most commonly reported fistulae of this type connect to the right ventricle but connections to the right atrium, pulmonary artery, and coronary sinus have also been described [21]. The functional significance of these communications depends on their number and amount of blood flow they conduct [22]. When there is significant shunting of blood under systemic pressure into the right side of the heart, pulmonary hypertension can develop and right heart failure may ensue. The case described above demonstrates fistulous communication of both right and left coronary arteries with the left ventricular cavity. Connections of this nature are much rarer than right-sided fistulae and only a handful of cases have been described in the world literature [21,24–29]. Reports

of myocardial ischemia, presumably from a "steal phenomenon," and congestive heart failure from a situation analogous to aortic valvular insufficiency and
left ventricular volume overload are some of the clinical consequences of such
communications [28,29]. In the case presented above, it is unlikely that her pre-
sentation to the hospital was related to her fistulae in view of her age at presen-
tation, the lack of recurrent symptoms, and the relatively small volume of blood
traversing the fistulae. However, the presenting symptoms prompted angiographic study, leading to the discovery of the apparently asymptomatic fistulae.
No standard method of treating symptomatic patients exists, although various
surgical approaches for fistula ligation have been described [21,22].

Pathology of persistent myocardial sinusoids in human hearts

The description of the myocardial sinusoids by Wearn in the 1930s has never re-
ally been challenged by using the modern techniques of imaging available
today. Despite this, there is little or no reference to the presence of myocardial sinusoids in the normal human heart in modern textbooks of histology [30]. As
cardiac surgeons are aware, the left ventricular myocardium does not look or
feel "spongy," nor does it give such an appearance on ventriculogram or on
echocardiogram. However, there are some rare pathologic conditions in which
these conditions, prominent in fetal hearts, persist into adulthood.

Myocardial sinusoids in association with complex congenital heart defects

Persistence of embryonic blood supply has been documented in neonates with
complex congenital cardiac defects. The most commonly described defect is
pulmonary atresia with intact ventricular septum [12,31,32]. It has been proposed that the excessively high right ventricular pressure associated with this
condition leads to the persistence of myocardial sinusoids that are prevalent
during early fetal development. In certain instances, these sinusoids persist as
an outflow for right ventricular blood through communications of the sinusoids
with the coronary arteries. The outflow route is possible when the right ventricle
pressure exceeds the systemic pressure present in the coronary arteries [13]. One
study described some of the adverse effects on left ventricular function from
persisting right ventricular sinusoids communicating with the left anterior descending coronary artery (LAD) [13]. The study showed significantly poorer
function of the left ventricular apex in cases of pulmonary atresia with intact
ventricular septum that had sinusoidal communications with the LAD, compared with similar cases that did not retain such communications. These findings were attributed to the mixing of deoxygenated right ventricular blood with
the LAD blood supplying the left ventricular apex. An analogous condition to
pulmonary atresia with the persistence of sinusoids has been described on the
left side of the heart in a case of aortic atresia with hypoplastic left ventricle [14].
Again, the sinusoids persisted as an outflow pathway for left ventricular blood
back into the right side of the circulation. The persistence of functional sinusoids

in this case was again attributed to abnormally high left ventricular pressure during development.

Non-compaction of ventricular myocardium as an isolated entity

The above examples of ventricular non-compaction associated with complex cardiac defects make it difficult to determine the effects that can be attributed solely to a persisting embryonic circulation. However, several small series of patients exist in the literature with persistence of heavy traveculations of the left ventricle as an isolated anomaly [20,33–37]. This condition has been termed isolated non-compaction of left ventricular myocardium. There is a wide range of severity of this condition, which probably leads to underestimating its prevalence. Patients present with clinical syndromes ranging from being asymptomatic to having severe heart failure, thromboembolic events, and potentially fatal ventricular arrhythmias [20]. Dusek *et al.* [17] have suggested that hypoxia in the subendocardium during development may lead to non-compaction of the ventricle leading to incomplete transformation of the fetal vasculature to the adult type. The etiology of congestive heart failure in these patients is not entirely clear but may be related to the inefficiency of such myocardial perfusion patterns, prevalent in cold-blooded animals, now confronted with the increased metabolic demands of warm-blooded mammals. There is an increased risk of thromboembolic events in this population and both systemic and pulmonary emboli have been reported [20,33]. Ventricular thrombi may form in the deep trabecular recesses and the problem may be exacerbated by the worsening ventricular function when the heart begins to fail. Ventricular arrhythmias found in this group of patients may be a consequence of worsening left ventricular function or a result of the scarring and fibrosis that are associated with some of the deep trabeculae [33].

Echocardiography is the diagnostic modality of choice. Ritter *et al.* [33] recently used the following criteria for diagnosis of non-compaction: the absence of any coexisting cardiac anomalies; prominent and excessive trabecular meshwork; and intertrabecular spaces perfused from the ventricular cavity, as visualized on color Doppler imaging.

Treatment for this rare and often misdiagnosed condition consists of management of the sequelae (heart failure, arrhythmias, and thrombi). In severe cases, heart transplantation could be the treatment of choice. The majority of patients remain asymptomatic and require no specific treatment other than careful follow-up by a physician who is aware of this entity.

Conclusions

The presence of myocardial sinusoids in the normal adult myocardium had been a subject of controversy for many years. Surgeons have applied this concept to devise treatments targeted at patients with ischemic heart disease. These surgical interventions included the Vineberg procedure and, more recently, transmyocardial laser revascularization (TMR). The substantial developments in the lasers designed for TMR were originally based on the concept that TMR channels made with the laser would stay open longer than channels made with a needle. These open channels would then direct blood from the ventricular cavity into the myocardial sinusoidal network, thus perfusing ischemic myocardium. The evidence suggests that such sinusoids do not even exist in the mature human heart.

We have reviewed the developmental anatomy of the mammalian heart through the early stages of the spongy reptilian-like myocardium and sinusoidal network to the mature compacted myocardium perfused solely by the coronary arteries. We have described instances where the early myocardial vascular pattern persists, in the form of coronary–ventricular fistulae, persisting sinusoids, and non-compaction of the ventricular myocardium. These are rare pathologic conditions and are often associated with adverse clinical outcomes. If treatments such as TMR are indeed clinically useful, we need to seek alternative explanations for their mechanisms of action in order to optimize them as effective therapies [15,16,38].

References

1 Wearn JT, Mettier SR, Klumpp TG, Zschiesche LJ. The nature of the vascular communications between the coronary arteries and the chambers of the heart. *Am Heart J* 1933;**9**: 143–64.

2 Vineberg AM, Miller D. Development of an anastomosis between the coronary vessels and a transplanted internal mammary artery. *Can Med Assoc J* 1947;**56**:609–14.

3 Vineberg AM, Buller W. Technical factors which favour mammary-coronary anastomosis: report of forty-five cases of human coronary artery disease thus treated. *J Thorac Surg* 1955;**30**:411–35.

4 Massimo C, Boffi L. Myocardial revascularisation by a new method of carrying blood directly from the left ventricular cavity into the coronary circulation. *J Thorac Surg* 1957;**34**:257–64.

5 Sen PK, Udwadia TE, Kinare SG, Parulkar GB. Transmyocardial acupuncture: a new approach to myocardial revascularization. *J Thorac Cardiovasc Surg* 1965;**50**:181–9.

6 Pifarre R, Jasuja ML, Lynch RD, Neville WE. Myocardial revascularization by transmyocardial acupuncture: a physiologic impossibility. *J Thorac Cardiovasc Surg* 1969;**58**:424–31.

7 Favaloro R, Effler DB, Groves LK, Sones FM Jr, Fergusson BJG. Myocardial revascularization by internal mammary artery implant procedures: clinical experience. *J Thorac Cardiovasc Surg* 1967;**54**:359–70.

8 Green GE, Stertzer SH, Reppert EH. Coronary artery bypass grafts. *Ann Thorac Surg* 1968;**5**:443–50.

9 Mirhoseini M, Cayton MM. Revascularization of the heart by laser. *J Microsurg* 1981;**2**:253–60.

10 Miroseini M, Shelgikar S, Cayton MM. New concepts in revascularization of the myocardium. *Ann Thorac Surg* 1988;**45**:415–20.

11 Tsang JC-C, Chiu RC-J. The phantom of "myocardial sinusoids": a historical reappraisal. *Ann Thorac Surg* 1995;**60**:1831–5.

12 Lauer RM, Fink HP, Petry EL, Dunn MI, Diehl AM. Angiographic demonstration of intramyocardial sinusoids in pulmonary-valve atresia with intact ventricular septum and hypoplastic right ventricle. *N Engl J Med* 1964;**271**:68–72.

13 Huasorf G, Gravinghoff L, Keck EW. Effects of persisting myocardial sinusoids on left ventricular performance in pulmonary atresia with intact ventricular septum. *Eur Heart J* 1987;**8**:291–6.

14 Raghib G, Bloemendaal RD, Kanjuh VI, Edwards JE. Aortic atresia and premature closure of foramen ovale: myocardial sinusoids and coronary ateriovenous fistula serving as an outflow channel. *Am Heart J* 1965;**70**:476–80.

15 Pelletier MP, Giaid A, Sivaraman S, *et al*. Angiogenesis and growth factor expression in a model of transmyocardial revascularization. *Ann Thorac Surg* 1998;**66**:12–8.

16 Chu V, Giaid A, Kuang J-Q, *et al*. Angiogenic response to transmyocardial revascularization (TMR): laser versus mechanical punctures [abstract]. Presented at the 35th Annual Meeting of the Society of Thoracic Surgeons, San Antonio, Texas. Jan 25–27, 1999.

17 Dusek J, Ostadal B, Duskova J. Postnatal persistence of spondy myocardium with embryonic blood supply. *Arch Pathol* 1975;**99**:312–7.

18 Grant RT. Development of the cardiac coronary vessels in the rabbit. *Heart* 1926;**13**:261–71.

19 Rychter Z, Jirasek JE, Rychterova V, Uher J. Vascularization of heart in human embryo: location and shape of non-vascularized part of cardiac wall. *Folia Morphol* 1975;**23**:88–96.

20 Chin TK, Perloff JK, Williams RG, Jue K, Mohrmann R. Isolated noncompaction of left ventricular myocardium: a study of eight cases. *Circulation* 1990;**82**:507–13.

21 McNamara JJ, Gross RE. Congenital coronary artery fistula. *Surgery* 1969;**65**:59–69.

22 De Nef JJE, Varghese PJ, Losekoot G. Congenital coronary artery fistula: analysis of 17 cases. *Br Heart J* 1971;**33**:857–62.

23 Rose AG. Multiple coronary arterioventricular fistulae. *Circulation* 1978;**58**:178–80.

24 Vogelbach KH, Edmiston WA, Stenson RE. Coronary artery–left ventricular communications: a report of two cases and review of the literature. *Cathet Cardiovasc Diagn* 1979;**5**:159–67.

25 Chia BL, Chan ALK, Tan LKA, Ng RAL, Chiang SP. Coronary artery–left ventricular fistula. *Cardiology* 1981;**68**:167–79.

26 Yokawa S, Watanabe H, Kurosaki M. Asymptomatic left and right coronary artery–left ventricular fistula in an elderly patient with a diastolic murmur only. *Int Cardiol* 1989;**25**:244–6.

27 Black IW, Loo CKC, Allan RM. Multiple coronary artery–left ventricular fistulae: clinical, angiographic, and pathologic findings. *Cathet Cardiovasc Diagn* 1991;**23**:133–5.

28 Duckworth F, Mukharji J, Vertrovec GW. Diffuse coronary to left ventricular communications: an unusual case of demonstrable ischaemia. *Cathet Cardiovasc Diagn* 1987;**13**:133–7.

29 Sheikhzadeh A, Stierle U, Langbehn AF, Thoran P, Diederich KW. Generalised coronary arterio-systemic (left ventricular) fistula: case report and review of the literature. *Jpn Heart J* 1986;**27**:533–44.

30 Billingham ME. Normal Heart. In: Sternberg SS (ed.) *History for Pathologists*, 2nd edn. Philadelphia: Lippencott-Raven, 1997: 745–60.

31 Grant RT. Unusual anomaly of coronary vessels in malformed heart of child. *Heart* 1926;**13**:273–83.

32 Williams RR, Kent GB Jr, Edwards JE. Anomalous cardiac blood vessel communicating with right ventricle: observations in case of pulmonary atresia with intact ventricular septum. *Arch Pathol* 1951;**52**:480–7.

33 Ritter M, Oechslin E, Sutsch G, *et al*. Isolated noncompaction of the myocardium in adults. *Mayo Clin Proc* 1997;**72**:26–31.

34 Shah CP, Nagi KS, Thakur RK, Boughner DR, Xie B. Spongy left ventricular myocardium in an adult. *Tex Heart Inst J* 1998;**25**:150–1.

35 Jenni R, Goebel N, Tartini R, *et al*. Persisting myocardial sinusoids of both ventricles as an isolated anomaly: echocardiographic, angiographic, and pathologic anatomical findings. *Cardiovasc Intervent Radiol* 1986;**9**:127–31.

36 Reynen K, Bachmann K, Singer H. Spongy myocardium. *Cardiology* 1997;**88**:601–2.

37 Steiner I, Hurbecky J, Pleskot J, Kokstejn Z. Persistence of spongy myocardium with embryonic blood supply in an adult. *Cardiovasc Pathol* 1996;**5**:47–53.

38 Malekan R, Reynolds C, Kelley S, *et al*. Angiogenesis in transmyocardial laser revascularization: a non-specific response to injury. *Circulation* 1997;**96**(Suppl 1):564.

CHAPTER 13

Remodeling of the intrinsic cardiac nervous system following chronic transmyocardial laser therapy

J Andrew Armour

Introduction

As is depicted throughout this volume, many patients with anatomically diffuse, end-stage coronary artery disease who are not amenable to standard revascularization procedures typically suffer from intractable angina despite the application of medical therapy. Several prospective studies have demonstrated that the creation of multiple transmural channels in the ischemic ventricle by means of a laser (transmyocardial laser revascularization [TMR]) provides symptomatic relief to patients experiencing such refractory angina [1–4].

Channels produced through the wall of an ischemic ventricular region by such a procedure were initially thought to remain patent after the procedure, thereby providing pathways for oxygenated blood to flow from the chamber into the affected myocardium [2,5–7]. However, with the subsequent demonstration that such channels remain patent for only a short period of time, this theory has been challenged [8–10]. Thus, alternative hypotheses have been promulgated in order to account for the efficacy of TMR. Among them is the suggestion that lesions produced through the left ventricular wall by means of a laser result in non-specific damage to tissues adjacent to the track so produced that may involve local neural tissues [11].

Cardiac neuronal hierarchy in the setting of acute TMR

Overview

It has been hypothesized that the tracts produced through the ventricular wall by means of laser affect the function of adjacent sensory neurites and autonomic efferent postganglionic nerves and their terminals [9,11]. In such a scenario, local laser-induced injury would obtund the capacity of regional ventricular sensory neurites to transduce the ischemic myocardium to central neurons via cardiac afferent neurons in nodose and dorsal root ganglia. As a consequence of their inability to transduce the ischemic myocardium to central neurons, symptomatic relief would be achieved [9].

On the other hand, if transmural laser channels damage adjacent efferent axons arising from more centrally located sympathetic efferent postganglionic neuronal somata then their ability to enhance regional ventricular contractility caudal to the sites of injury would become reduced [5,6]. Such local sympathetic efferent postganglionic axonal denervation would, in turn, minimize increased demands placed on the ischemic myocardium when the sympathetic nervous system becomes activated during the stress of exercise, for instance [9,11]. That neuronally induced enhancement of regional ventricular contractility may be held in check following TMR represents another mechanism whereby this procedure might influence ischemic ventricular function and indirectly the perception of an altered ventricular milieu.

Cardiac neuronal hierarchy

It has been proposed that the cardiac nervous system comprises a hierarchy of central and peripheral interconnecting neurons that are in constant communication with one another to match cardiac output to body demands [12]. The final common integrator of cardiac sensory to motor neuron transduction is represented by the nervous system intrinsic to the heart [13]. The intrinsic cardiac nervous system is made up of collections of ganglia and interconnecting nerves that form discrete atrial and ventricular ganglionated plexuses [14,15]. Each atrial and ventricular ganglionated plexus contains afferent neurons, cholinergic and adrenergic efferent neurons, as well as interconnecting local circuit neurons [12]. The latter population of neurons projects axons to neurons either within their ganglia or outside of their respective ganglia, that is to neurons throughout their intrinsic cardiac ganglionated plexus as well as to neurons in other intrinsic cardiac ganglionated plexuses [16] and more centrally located extracardiac ganglia [12]. Thus, the presence of local circuit neurons is relevant for the transduction of cardiac sensory information to cardiac motor neurons. Because of the complex functional connectivity of the intrathoracic nervous system, each neuronal population within it needs to be tested selectively.

Cardiac afferent neurons

Cardiac afferent neurons are located in various intrinsic cardiac ganglionated plexuses, in intrathoracic extracardiac ganglia, as well as in nodose and dorsal root ganglia [17–19]. Cardiac sensory neurons provide inputs to second-order neurons located at each level of the cardiac neuronal hierarchy [12]. Thus, any alteration in the cardiac milieu is transduced by these afferent neurons to intrathoracic and central second-order neurons to generate peripheral (intrathoracic) and central cardiac-cardiovascular reflexes of varying latencies [20].

The sensory neurites (nerve endings) associated with cardiac chemosensory neurons transduce multiple chemicals liberated into their local interstitium from adjacent myocardial and other cells [21]. As the sensory neurites associated with some afferent neurons are located in the ventricular epicardium, epicardial application of a chemical modifies the activity generated by such neurons in a direct manner [21]. One such chemical that does so without eliciting tachyphylaxis is the Na^+-channel modifier veratridine. Thus, veratridine can be applied repeatedly to a cardiac sensory field in order to test the capacity of cardiac afferent neurons to transduce the local chemical milieu before and after altering cardiac status.

Sympathetic or parasympathetic efferent postganglionic neurons

Sympathetic or parasympathetic efferent postganglionic neurons that innervate various ventricular regions can be selectively activated by electrically stimulating decentralized stellate ganglia or the cervical vagosympathetic complexes, respectively [22–24]. As cardiac adrenergic and cholinergic efferent postganglionic neurons possess nicotinic receptors, both populations can also be activated by systemic administration of nicotine to test their capacity to modulate the heart [22].

Local cicuit neurons

The function of intrinsic cardiac local circuit neurons can be assessed by a process of exclusion. Most neurons within the intrinsic cardiac ganglia do not receive direct inputs from cardiovascular sensory neurites [15,25,26], nor do they receive direct inputs from extracardiac motor (efferent) neurons [12]. As such, most intrinsic cardiac neurons receive multisynaptic inputs from medullary (parasympathetic) and intrathoracic (sympathetic) efferent neurons, as well as from cardiopulmonary afferent neurons [12]. As they receive multisynaptic inputs from these sources, it has been proposed that this population functions as interneurons [12,13]. Because most of them interact not only with adjacent neurons in their ganglia, but also with neurons in other intrinsic cardiac [26] and intrathoracic extracardiac ganglia [25], they have been identified as local circuit neurons [12,13].

Local inotropic responses

In order to assess the contractile function of the myocardium in which multiple transmural canals have been produced, local inotropic responses induced in a treated zone following exogenous administration of a β-adrenergic receptor agonist can be compared with augmentor responses so elicited in adjacent unaffected ventricular tissues by means of local implantable pressure sensors [27].

Cardiac nervous system following acute TMR

Cardiac afferent neurons

Kwong *et al.* [9], by applying high doses of bradykinin to the ventricular epicardium overlying the treated ventricle before and after TMR and analyzing the cardiovascular reflexes so elicited, concluded that TMR renders sensory neurites in the affected myocardium non-functional. However, direct assessment of the capacity of cardiac afferent neurons to transduce the local milieu of treated ventricular tissues found that such is not the case [27]. The capacity of intrinsic cardiac afferent neurons to transduce the chemical milieu in the affected myocardium was similar to sensory transduction in unaffected ventricular regions, as well as that identified in normal canine hearts [25,26]. Presumably, that is because individual cardiac afferent neurons are associated with multiple sensory neurites (nerve endings) that are diffusely spread throughout a ventricular region – the sensory field of that afferent neuron [17–19,28]. This makes it extremely unlikely that the production of a relatively limited number of small diameter holes through the wall of a ventricle would affect enough of them such that their capacity to transduce the local cardiac milieu to their associated somata becomes obtunded. In other words, the transmural lesions produced by TMR would not have affected sufficient numbers of the sensory neurites associated with individual cardiac afferent neurons to noticeably affect their ability to transduce the treated milieu.

Cardiac efferent neurons

It has been found that myocardial tissue tyrosine hydroxylase immunoreactivity, an indirect measure of sympathetic efferent postganglionic axonal density, becomes reduced in ventricular regions subjected to TMR [11]. By implication, this should result in regional sympathetic efferent neuronal denervation. However, direct assessment of the capacity of cardiac sympathetic efferent neurons to influence mechanical events within and caudal to the treated myocardium (and, for that matter, in the untreated ventricle) demonstrated that TMR does not affect that capacity [27]. In the setting of acute TMR, cardiac adrenergic efferent neurons continue to enhance regional ventricular dynamics to degrees found before its application; their augmentor capacity matched that identified in the untreated ventricular regions. This occurred whether these efferent neurons were activated electrically or chemically [27].

Acute TMR does not alter the contractile behavior of the effected ventricular wall either [27]. Systemic administration of the β-adrenergic agonist isoproterenol enhanced intramyocardial systolic pressure similarly in treated and untreated left ventricular regions. Electrical stimulation of parasympathetic efferent preganglionic axons also induced similar myocardial contractile suppressor responses in acutely treated and untreated left ventricular regions. Taken together, these data demonstrate that TMR does not obtund the capacity of extracardiac autonomic efferent neurons to regulate regional ventricular function immediately following the initiation of TMR.

Local circuit neurons

Much of the information transduced by the intrinsic cardiac nervous system to cardiac motor neurons that arises from cardiac sensory neurons, as well as from more centrally located autonomic efferent neurons, depends on the presence of intrinsic cardiac local circuits neurons. As these local circuit neurons transduce both centripetal and centrifugal information, it has been proposed that they act collectively as a low pass filter [12,13]. As such they may perform a smoothing function in the presence of excessive inputs secondary to regional ventricular ischemia [29]; otherwise, excessive activation of cardiac motor neurons may lead to arrhythmia formation [30]. The creation of multiple laser channels through the wall of the left ventricle does not alter the capacity of intrinsic cardiac local circuit neurons to transduce cardiac sensory information to intrinsic cardiac motor neurons in the acute setting [27], nor does it affect their capacity to transduce inputs arising from central autonomic efferent neurons. This population of neurons also responds normally to exogenously administered chemicals such as nicotine or angiotensin II. Taken together, these data indicate that the creation of multiple channels through the ventral wall of the left ventricle does not alter the capacity of afferent, local circuit, and efferent neurons within the intrinsic cardiac nervous system to regulate regional ventricular function in the acute setting.

Cardiac neuronal hierarchy in the setting of chronic TMR

Recent evidence indicates that TMR imparts delayed remodeling of the intrinsic cardiac nervous system within a month after its instigation in a non-ischemic canine model [31]. Removal of inputs to this nervous system from more centrally located neurons also remodels its capacity to influence cardiodynamics in a chronic [32,34] but not acute setting [22]. Such remodeling occurs in a very selective manner, similar to that which occurs early on during the evolution of tachycardia-induced heart failure (32,33,34). In other words, the capacity of intrinsic cardiac nervous system to transduce the cardiac milieu to cardiac efferent neurons appears to be susceptible to altered cardiac status over time.

Cardiomyocyte function

One month after initiating TMR, exogenous administration of a β-adrenoceptor agonist enhanced left ventricular intramyocardial systolic pressure in the treated zone in a manner similar to that of unaffected ventricular regions or, for that matter, of control animals [22]. As both affected and unaffected ventricular regions responded similarly to such an intervention, it appears that chronic TMR does not modify the capacity of ventricular myocytes to generate contractile force. Furthermore, ventricular zones subjected to TMR do not display wall motion abnormalities (as assessed by echocardiographic analysis). These data indicate TMR does not depress regional ventricular contractile function significantly over time.

Cardiac afferent neurons

When the sodium-channel modifying agent veratridine is applied to sensory neurites in a ventricular zone that had been subjected to TMR 1 month previously, their associated intrinsic cardiac afferent neuronal somata behaved robustly. As a matter of fact, their responsiveness matched that of sensory neurons transducing untreated ventricular regions in such preparations [32,33], as well as that identified following acute application of TMR [27]. The sensory neurites in ventricular regions subjected to chronic TMR also transduce their local milieu in a fashion similar to that displayed by cardiac afferent neurons in normal animals [21]. As ventricular sensory neurites transduce the milieu of a ventricular zone exposed to long-term TMR normally, it appears that this form of therapy does not alter the transduction properties of cardiac afferent neurons in a chronic setting.

Cardiac efferent neurons

Stellate ganglion stimulation induces the same degree of ventricular augmentation in ventricular zones treated the previous month with TMR as occurs in untreated ventricular regions [31]. Furthermore, such responsiveness matches that identified in normal ventricles during sympathetic efferent neuronal activation [22]. The same holds true with respect to the capacity of cholinergic efferent neurons to suppress local ventricular intramyocardial systolic pressure in the chronic TMR setting [31]. Together, these data indicate that centrally located autonomic efferent preganglionic neurons exert normal control over long-term TMR-treated ventricular tissues.

Intrinsic cardiac local circuit neurons

However, the capacity of intrinsic cardiac local circuit neurons to transduce information arising from cardiac sensory neurons to cardiac motor neurons remodels in the setting of chronic TMR. One month after producing multiple channels through the ventral wall of the left ventricle, right atrial local circuit neurons proved to be insensitive to two neurochemical agonists that exert potent agonist activity on their behavior in normal preparations [12].

Exogenously administered nicotine normally activates populations of intrinsic cardiac neurons such that rapid cardiac parasympathetic postganglionic neuronal excitation is initiated that is accompanied by bradycardia and ventricular force suppression [22,27]. Cardiac sympathetic efferent postganglionic neuronal activation follows which results in the subsequent enhancement of cardiac indices [22]. Despite the fact that both populations of autonomic efferent neurons respond normally to systemic administration of nicotine in the acute setting of TMR (see above), they proved to be unresponsive to nicotine in the chronic setting of TMR. This occurred even when the dose of nicotine tested was four times greater than that required to elicit maximal heart rate and ventricular inotropic responses in normal preparations [22,31].

The same held true with respect to exogenously administered angiotensin II. When angiotensin II was administered in doses that excite intrinsic cardiac local circuit neurons to induce augmentor responses in normal preparations, no neuronal or cardiac responses were elicited in the chronic TMR setting. These data have been interpreted as indicating that TMR obtunds the capacity of nicotine and angiotensin II sensitive intrinsic cardiac regulatory neurons to affect cardiodynamics over time after its application [31].

In the chronic setting of TMR, nicotine failed to activate neurons such that intramyocardial systolic pressures in both the treated and unaffected ventricular regions did not increase; nor was heart rate affected [31]. Because that happened without any loss in the capacity of ventricular myocytes to respond to β-adrenoceptor agonists or extracardiac sympathetic efferent neuronal inputs, these data support the hypothesis that remodeling of the processing of cardiac sensory information within the cardiac neuronal hierarchy occurs in such a state. That such remodeling involves selective components of the cardiac neuronal hierarchy is evident from the observation that the responsiveness of intrinsic cardiac afferent and efferent neurons appears to be relatively unaffected subsequent to TMR. On the other hand, that chronic TMR affects the capacity of its local circuit neurons to transduce cardiac sensory information to influence cardiac indices does result in considerable remodeling of the overall function of the cardiac neuroaxis.

Perspectives

In the chronic setting, TMR remodels the final common processor of cardiac centrifugal and centripetal information by apparently obtunding the function of its local circuit neurons that transduce ventricular stress to cardiomotor neurons. It has been reported that while many patients receive symptomatic improvement soon after TMR, peak anginal relief is usually achieved 3–6 months after its induction [1,2,4]. That remodeling of selective components within the intrinsic cardiac nervous system takes time to occur following application of TMR to a region of the left ventricle may account, in part, for the delayed efficacy that this form of therapy affords some individuals.

If indeed such is the case, this therapy may act to stabilize inputs to cardiac motor neurons in pathologic states. First, the consequence of remodeling the capacity of intrinsic cardiac local circuit neurons to transduce excessive cardiac afferent neuronal information may result in less sensory information being transferred to central neurons, thereby reducing cardiac symptoms. Second, such remodeling may act to suppress cardio-cardiac reflexes initiated as a consequence of transducing the ischemic state. Reducing the enhancement of cardiac motor neuronal activity in such a state might minimize any propensity to cardiac arrhythmia formation arising as a consequence of excessive sympathetic efferent neuronal inputs to the heart [35].

What seems to be certain at present is that selective components of the intrinsic cardiac nervous system remodel over time following the induction of TMR. Stabilization of the capacity of intrinsic cardiac local circuit neurons to transduce regional ventricular ischemia can also be achieved by delivering high-frequency electrical stimuli to the cranial aspect of thoracic spinal cord [36]. The challenge remains to determine how this and other modes of therapy selectively target interactive neurons within the cardiac neuronal hierarchy to modify how the heart responds to stress.

Acknowledgments

The author gratefully acknowledges the support the Canada Institutes of Health Research and the Canadian Heart and Stroke Foundation.

References

1 Allen KB, Dowling RD, Fudge TL, *et al*. Comparison of transmyocardial revascularization with medical therapy in patients with refractory angina. *N Engl J Med* 1999;**341**:1029–36.

2 Frazier OH, March RJ, Horvath KA. Transmyocardial revascularization with a carbon dioxide laser in patients with end-stage coronary artery disease. *N Engl J Med* 1999;**341**: 1021–8.

3 Jones JW, Schmidt SE, Richman BW, *et al*. Holmium:YAG laser transmyocardial revascularization relieves angina and improves functional status. *Ann Thorac Surg* 1999;**67**: 1596–601.

4 Schofield PM, Sharples LD, Caine N, *et al*. Transmyocardial laser revascularization in patients with refractory angina: a randomized controlled trial. *Lancet* 1999;**353**:519–24.

5 Burkhoff D, Fisher PE, Apfelbaum M, *et al*. Histological appearance of transmyocardial laser channels after 4_ weeks. *Ann Thorac Surg* 1996;**61**:1532–6.

6 Fleischer KJ, Goldschmidt-Clermont PJ, Fonger JD, *et al*. One-month histological response to transmyocardial laser channels with molecular intervention. *Ann Thorac Surg* 1996; **62**:1051–8.

7 Gassler N, Wintzer H-O, Stubbe H-M, Wullbrand A, Helmchen U. Transmyocardial laser revascularization: histological features in human nonresponder myocardium. *Circulation* 1997;**95**:371–5.

8 Kohmoto T, Fisher PE, Gu A, *et al*. Physiology, histology, and 2-week morphology of acute transmyocardial channels made with a CO_2 laser. *Ann Thorac Surg* 1997;**63**:1275–83.

9 Kwong KF, Kanellopoulos GK, Nickols JC, *et al*. Transmyocardial laser treatment denervates canine myocardium. *J Thorac Cardiovasc Surg* 1997;**114**:883–90.

10 Whittaker P. Transmyocardial revascularization: the fate of myocardial channels. *Ann Thorac Surg* 1999;**68**:2376–82.

11 Al Sheikh T, Allen KB, Straka SP, *et al*. Cardiac sympathetic denervation after transmyocardial laser revascularization. *Circulation* 1999;**100**:135–40.

12 Armour JA. Anatomy and function of the intrathoracic neurons regulating the mammalian heart. In: Zucker IH, Gilmore JP (eds). *Reflex Control of the Circulation*. Boca Raton, FL: CRC Press, 1991: 1–37.

13 Ardell JL. Structure and function of mammalian intrinsic cardiac neurons. In: Armour JA, Ardell JL (eds). *Neurocardiology*. New York: Oxford University Press, 1994: 95–115.

14 Armour JA, Murphy DA, Yuan B-X, MacDonald S, Hopkins DA. Anatomy of the human intrinsic cardiac nervous system. *Anat Record* 1997;**297**:289–98.

15 Yuan B-X, Ardell JL, Hopkins DA, Armour JA. Gross and microscopic anatomy of canine intrinsic cardiac neurons. *Anat Record* 1994;**239**:75–87.

16 Randall DC, Brown DR, McGuirt AS, *et al*. Interactions within the intrinsic cardiac nervous system contribute to chronotropic regulation. *Am J Physiol* 2003;**285**:R1066–75.

17 Armour JA. Physiological behavior of thoracic cardiovascular receptors. *Am J Physiol* 1973;**225**:177–85.

18 Coleridge JCG, Coleridge HM. Chemoreflex regulation of the heart. In: Berne RM, Sperelakis N, Geiger S (eds). *Handbook of Physiology, Section 2: The Cardiovascular System*. Bethesda: American Physiological Society, 1979: 653–76.

19 Thorén P. Role of cardiac vagal c-fibers in cardiovascular control. *Rev Physiol Biochem Pharmacol* 1979;**86**:1–94.

20 Armour JA. Instant-to-instant reflex cardiac regulation. *Cardiology* 1976;**61**:309–28.

21 Thompson GW, Horackova M, Armour JA. Chemotransduction properties of nodose ganglion cardiac afferent neurons in guinea-pigs. *Am J Physiol* 2000;**279**:R433–9.

22 Murphy DA, O'Blenes S, Hanna BD, Armour JA. Capacity of intrinsic cardiac neurons to modify the acutely autotransplanted mammalian heart. *J Heart Lung Transplant* 1994;**13**:847–56.

23 Randall WC. Efferent sympathetic innervation of the heart. In: Armour JA, Ardell JL (eds). *Neurocardiology.* New York: Oxford University Press, 1994: 77–94.

24 Randall WC, Armour JA. Regional vagosympathetic control of the heart. *Am J Physiol* 1974;**227**:444–52.

25 Armour JA, Collier K, Kember G, Ardell JL. Differential selectivity of cardiac neurons in separate intrathoracic ganglia. *Am J Physiol* 1998;**274**:R939–49.

26 Thompson GW, Collier K, Ardell JL, Kember G, Armour JA. Functional interdependence of neurons in a single canine intrinsic cardiac ganglionated plexus. *J Physiol* 2000;**528**:561–71.

27 Hirsch GM, Thompson GW, Arora RC, *et al.* Transmyocardial laser revascularization does not denervate the canine heart. *Ann Thorac Surg* 1999;**68**:460–9.

28 Foreman RD, Blair RW, Holmes, HR, Armour JA. Correlation of activity generated by sympathetic afferent ventricular mechanosensory neurites with sensory field deformation in the normal and ischemic myocardium. *Am J Physiol* 1999;**276**:R976–89.

29 Kember GC, Fenton GA, Collier K, Armour JA. Stochastic resonance in a hysteretic population of cardiac neurons. *Physical Rev E* 2000;**61**:1816–24.

30 Huang MH, Wolf SG, Armour JA. Ventricular arrhythmias induced by chemically modified intrinsic cardiac neurons. *Cardiovasc Res* 1994;**28**:636–42.

31 Arora RC, Hirsch G, Hirsch K, Armour JA. Transmyocardial laser revascularization remodels the intrinsic cardiac nervous system in a chronic setting. *Circulation* 2001;**104**:I101–20.

32 Arora RC, Cardinal R, Smith FM, *et al.* Tachycardia induced heart failure remodels the intrinsic cardiac nervous system. *Am J Physiol* 2003;**285**:R1212–23.

33 Tallaj J, Wei C-C, Hanks GH, *et al.* β_1-adrenergic receptor blockade attenuates angiotensin II mediated catecholamine release into the cardiac interstitium in mitral regurgitation. *Circ* 2003;**108**:225–30.

34 Murphy DA, Thompson GW, Ardell JL, *et al.* The heart reinnervates after transplantation. *Ann Thorac Surg* 2000;**69**:1769–81.

35 Cardinal R, Scherlag BJ, Vermeulen M, Armour JA. Distinct activation patterns of idioventricular rhythms and sympathetically-induced ventricular tachycardias in dogs with atrioventricular block. *Pace* 1992;**15**:1300–16.

36 Linderoth B, Foreman RD. Physiology of spinal cord stimulation: review and update. *Neuromodulation* 1999;**2**:150–64.

Index

Note: Page numbers in *italic* refer to figures and/or tables